THE VAGINA CHRONICLES

Breaking Myths and Fostering Empowerment

Betty Iliadis

Free Publishing

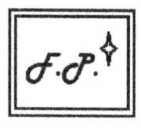

Copyright © 2024 Paraskevi Iliadou

All rights reserved

No part of this book may be reproduced, or stored in a retrieval system, or transmitted in any form or by any means, electronic, mechanical, photocopying, recording, or otherwise, without express written permission of the copyright owner.

This publication is designed to provide accurate and authoritative information in regard to the subject matter covered. It is sold with the understanding that neither the author nor the publisher is engaged in rendering legal, investment, accounting or other professional services. While the publisher and author have used their best efforts in preparing this work, they make no representations or warranties with respect to the accuracy or completeless of the contents of this book and specifically disclaim any implied warranties of merchantability or fitness for a particular purpose. No warranty may be created or extended by sales representatives or written sales materials. The advice and strategies contained herein may not be suitable for your situation. You should consult with a professional when appropriate. Neither the publisher nor the author shall be liable for any loss or profit or any other commercial damages, including but not limited to special, incidental, consequential, personal or other damages.

Book cover created on Canva by the author.

First edition
2024

Dedicated to all women who endured physical, psychological, and emotional pain and emerged even stronger.

CONTENTS

Title Page	
Copyright	
Dedication	
Preface	
Introduction	1
About Vagina	6
Prejudices and Myths	17
The Toilet Rule	20
Hair removal and vagina	22
Menstruation and Period-Poverty	26
MENOPAUSE	33
Sensitive area and exercise	39
Vulvoplasty	43
Vaginal Bleaching	46
Controversial vaginal care Recommendations	49
part two	51
Female genital mutilation	54
Physical effects of FGM	72
Psychological effects of FGM	75
A GEOGRAPHICAL APPROACH OF FGM	78
AFRICA	80

ASIA-PACIFIC REGION	89
MIDDLE EAST	94
EUROPE	97
UNITED KINGDOM	103
FGM and the nhs	127
FGM-IS	130
MEASURES AGAINST FGM	133
part three	178
Menstrual Taboos	185
ACTIVISTS and AMNESTY INTERNATIONAL	194
CHHAUPADI	203
EPILOGUE	209
Reference List	213
Afterword	223
About The Author	225

PREFACE

In the intricate nature of human existence, there is a profound and enigmatic force that has captured hearts, inspired creativity and sparked countless conversations - the vagina. Often shrouded in mystery, burdened by misconceptions and subject to social taboos, thid remarkable part of the female anatomy has endured a complicated history of misunderstanding and oppression.

"TheVagina Chronicles : Breakig Myths and Fostering Empowerment" is a journey into the heart of womanhood - a celebration of resilience, strength, and power of knowledge. As we embark on this odyssey, let us cast aside the veils of silence and set about a quest to uncover the truths that have been obscured by socia norms and cultural myths.

In the following pages, we will navigate the maze of historical misconceptions and patriarchal constructs, dispelling the shadows that have obscured the innate power and beauty of the vagina. This is not just a collection of stories, but a manifesto for reclaiming autonomy, challenging stigmas, and fostering a sense of empowerment to each individual.

The Vagina Chronicles is an ode to diversity - recognising that every vagina has its own unique story to tell, a narrative shaped by personal experiences, cultural backgrounds, and the intersections of identity. Through personal narratives, expert knowledge and a wealth of information, we aim to cultivate an environment where knowledge becomes a tool of liberation and empowerment.

INTRODUCTION

I come from a middle-class family where the use of the word vagina was forbidden and associated with something obscene. While it's commonplace to articulate feelings of stomach discomfort or acknowledge a runny nose with ease, addressing any sensations related to the vagina tends to require delicate language. In our discussions, we readily navigate the complexities of our digestive system, yet when it comes to conversations about the female genitals, we often resort to euphemistic expressions such as 'scratch down there' or 'wash that area.' Alternatively, subtle gestures are employed instead of direct language.

During our time in school, we dedicated weeks to studying photosynthesis's intricacies, which I never quite grasped. Unfortunately, we never delved into the reproductive system because the school year concluded before we could cover it.

Our comprehension of our feminine essence was in complete disarray. Invariably, there were always those unconventional friends who held unique insights and discreetly shared them with us during our gatherings.

Amid these prevailing biases, we matured with a sense of guilt about our bodies and shame associated with our female identity. Anxiously, we sought to justify our absences to teachers during the "challenging days" and conceal any discomfort or stains on the back of our uniforms. The most poignant moments were when we had to navigate across a classroom to reach the teacher's desk for permission to visit the restroom during class, all while enduring the ironic glances of our peers, aware that we were the subject of ridicule.

I consistently ensure there's a sanitary pad in my bag, both for unexpected situations and, as my mother used to advise, to stay prepared. I also recall consistently experiencing a sense of discomfort whenever it was time for gynaecological examinations at the medical practice.

Undoubtedly, those experiences seem like the bygone years of my adolescence and youth, and fortunately, they are now a distant memory. In contemporary times, individuals can readily find comfort in the camaraderie of classmates during breaks, discussing pain or openly communicating about menstruation—akin to acknowledging a common headache.

However, the stark realisation hit me that what now seems natural and obvious to other women remains a recurring nightmare for many. I became acutely aware that millions of women worldwide endure torment and relinquish their womanhood in the name of religion, traditions, or morality—a morality that consistently works against them, jeopardising their lives and prevailing over them rather than being in their favour.

I've always struggled to comprehend how someone can become spiritually blind and inflict physical and mental harm on a being that carries the precious gift of life within it.

Throughout centuries, entrenched customs and traditions have inflicted profound wounds upon women's souls, stifled their emotions, and ruthlessly victimised innocent bodies, all for the perceived "crime" of being born female. This tragic narrative unfolds without clear culprits, leaving an elusive void that criminology refers to as the generative cause. The perpetuation of such harm lacks a definitive origin, perpetuating a cycle that continues to impact women across generations. Perhaps there is a shared cause—the vagina. The body part that grants and receives pleasure and satisfaction, and, simultaneously, triggers pain, isolation, and stigmatisation.

Is this part of the body truly to blame for the countless sorrows that millions of women have endured? Or is it the result of centuries-old male misogyny that has consistently demonised female existence? Since the earliest times, women have been perceived as a threat to men, blamed for leading them into sin and, in turn, enticing all of humanity. The persistence of male prejudice and complexes continues to dominate, upholding medieval practices aimed at controlling and subjugating women.

On the other hand, there's a perspective suggesting that the so-called "impostor syndrome" might have a generational impact, transmitted through female genes. Women who conform to traditions and unspoken rules may not necessarily do so because they genuinely believe in their own value. Instead, it could be driven by a yearning for social acceptance, surpassing their self-esteem and deterring them from rebelling against sexist practices that aim to subjugate and sacrifice them.

Regardless of the cause, any harmful action against the vagina—more than just a part of the female body but the ultimate expression of female sexuality—elicits strong opposition from me. It not only contradicts my values but also stirs up feelings of anger and frustration, not unfairly directed towards the opposite sex. Reflecting on the fact that over 8 billion people on the planet have entered the world through the vagina is sobering. This process is a fundamental aspect of the existence of approximately 3.8 billion women worldwide.

Drawing from the insights of the German psychoanalyst Karen Horney, a pioneer in feminist psychology and women's psychiatry, men may harbour "vagina envy" due to their inability to experience childbirth, urination, and masturbation in the unique ways that women can (Ruitenbeek, 1966).

ABOUT VAGINA

At this juncture, I refrain from an in-depth exploration of the anatomical and functional intricacies of the vagina. These details, widely recognised, are readily available to those with an interest in the subject.

Let's begin with the etymology of the Greek word for the vagina, which is "aidoio." It originates from the ancient Greek adjective "aidoios," signifying "worthy of respect" (Lidell *et al.*, n.d p. 64).

As we shift from considering something worthy of respect to deeming it taboo in society, this transformation remains inexplicable and undeniably demands a cultural re-evaluation.

Examining art throughout history helps illuminate the significance and respect accorded to the vagina. Notably, Palaeolithic sculpted figurines of Aphrodite, dating between 28,000 BC and 25,000 BC, emphasise the vagina, with the Venus of Willendorf figurine currently exhibited at the Natural History Museum in Vienna standing out.

While discussing the artistic representation of the vagina, it is essential to explore historical and contemporary perspectives. For instance, a 16th-century female statuette from a Nepalese temple prominently features the vagina, emphasising its significance through the characteristic posture of the body. Moreover, the stone yoni in the Cat Tien Hindu temple in Lam Dong, Vietnam, is noteworthy. In Sanskrit, "yoni" translates to female genitalia organs or vagina, but its meaning transcends the physical aspect, symbolising creativity on a religious or spiritual level. Moving into the modern era, the 20th and 21st centuries have seen notable artists, including Niki de Saint Phalle, Jean Tinguely, Megumi Igarashi, and Anish Kapoor, engage in the creation of artworks that depict the vagina. This artistic evolution reflects a broader societal shift in acknowledging and celebrating the feminine form, fostering a dynamic dialogue between historical representations and contemporary interpretations.

Left: The Venus of Willendorf (The Collector, 2022)

Right: The stone yoni (Wikimedia, 2007)

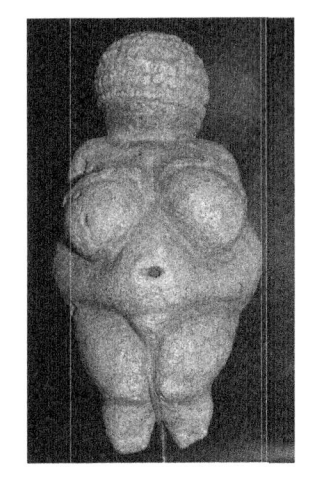

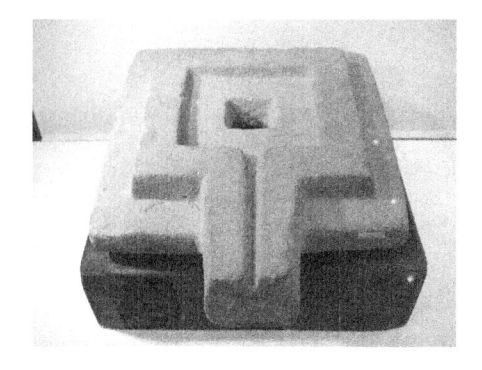

The Japanese visual artist and Manga designer Megumi Igarashi, also known by the pseudonym Rokudenashito, achieved acclaim for her visual representations of the vagina. Her work is a significant part of her advocacy against the societal taboo surrounding the depiction of female genitalia, drawing attention to the contrast with the more widely accepted depictions of male genitalia (Kendall, 2014). In her endeavour to create comprehensive artwork on the subject of the vagina, she took a bold step by constructing a Vagina Kayak shaped like a 3D scan of her own vagina, funding the project through crowdfunding. Following a police raid in Japan, many of her vagina-themed works were confiscated, and she faced accusations of violating Japanese morality laws.

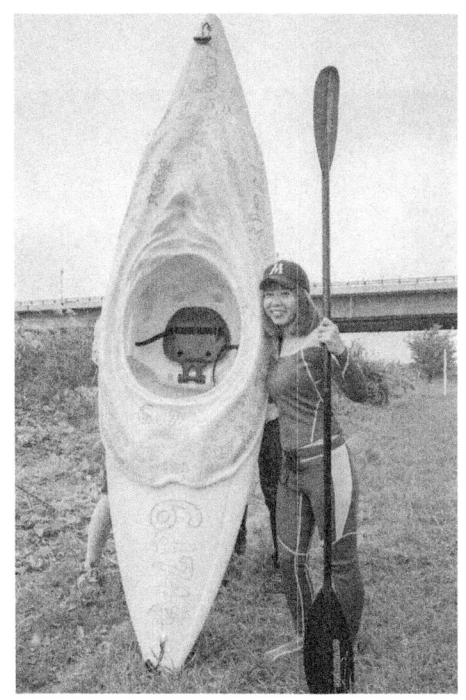

Megumi Igarashi, posing next to her vagina-shaped kayak (The London Free Press, 2014)

Arguably, the most iconic representation is Judy Chicago's feminist art piece, The Dinner Party. This installation features an isosceles triangle-shaped dinner table adorned with 39 vulva-shaped dishes, each bearing the name of a significant mythological or historical woman. Notable names like Empress Theodora of Byzantium, Virginia Woolf, Christine de Pisan, and Sojourner Truth are highlighted (the artwork is showcased at the Brooklyn Museum, specifically on the Heritage Floor).

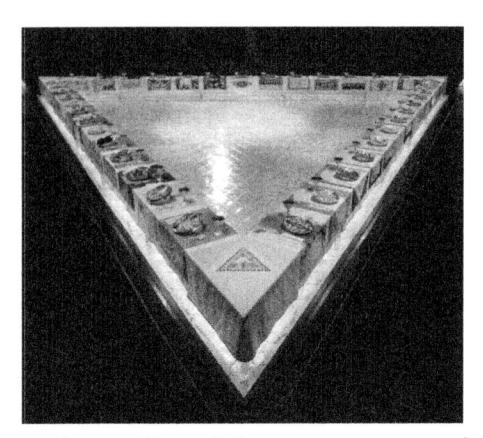

The Dinner Party (brooklynmuseum.org)

Recognising its utmost importance, we must acknowledge the significance of the inaugural Vagina Museum in London. It made its debut on November 16, 2019, and was subsequently relocated to Poyser Street, Bethnal Green, on April 11, 2023. This pioneering institution has a core mission: to foster open conversations about the vagina. By offering educational opportunities for both women and men, the museum seeks to demystify and destigmatize various aspects related to this integral part of the human anatomy.

The founder and director of the museum, Florence Schechter, explained her motivation behind the project in straightforward terms: "I discovered there was a penis museum in Iceland but no vagina equivalent anywhere else, so I decided to create one." (Lawford, 2023).

The mission of the museum is to:
1. Spread knowledge and raise awareness of gynaecological anatomy and health.
2. Give confidence to talk about issues surrounding gynaecological anatomy.
3. Erase the stigma around the body and gynaecological anatomy.
4. Act as a forum for feminism, women's rights, the LGBTQ+ community, and the intersex community.
5. Challenge heteronormative and cisnormative behaviour.
6. Promote intersectional, feminist, and trans-inclusive values.

In the realm of breaking societal taboos, this initiative strives to provide women with a sense of empowerment and the delight of belonging to a remarkable community.

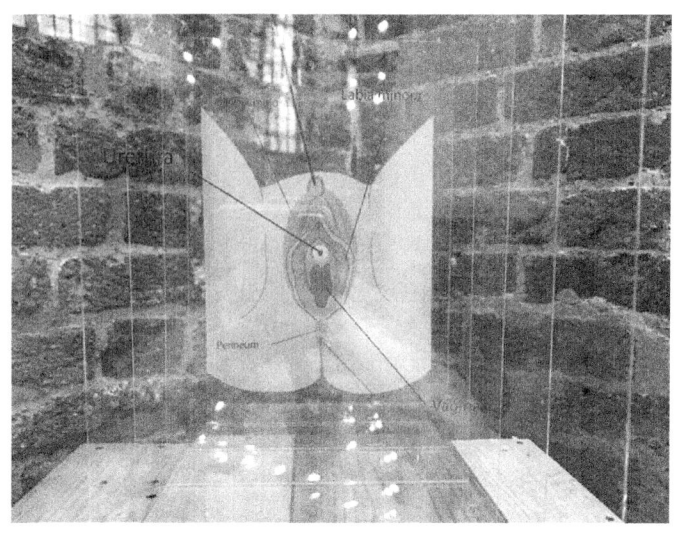

Model of female anatomy (Johnston, 2019).

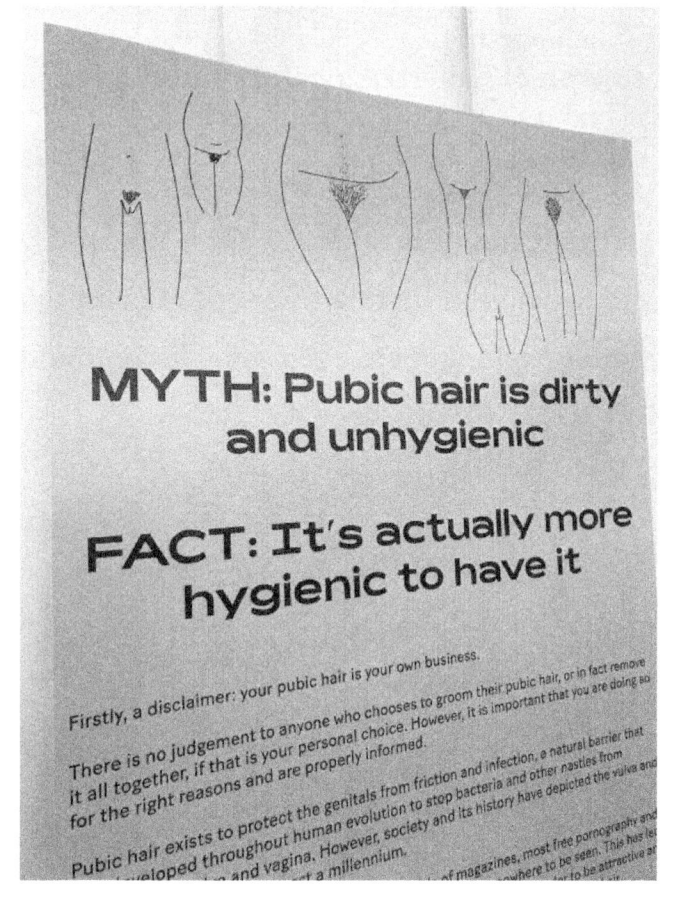

MYTH: Pubic hair is dirty and unhygienic

FACT: It's actually more hygienic to have it

Firstly, a disclaimer: your pubic hair is your own business.

There is no judgement to anyone who chooses to groom their pubic hair, or in fact remove it all together, if that is your personal choice. However, it is important that you are doing so for the right reasons and are properly informed.

Pubic hair exists to protect the genitals from friction and infection, a natural barrier that developed throughout human evolution to stop bacteria and other nasties from ... and vagina. However, society and its history have depicted the vulva and ... a millennium. ... of magazines, most free pornography and ... where to be seen. This has le... ... to be attractive a...

Message on pubic hair (Johnston, 2019).

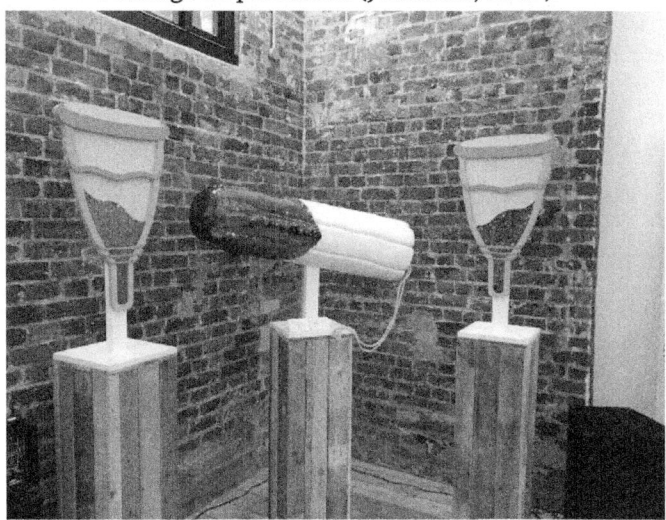

Artwork (Johnston, 2019).

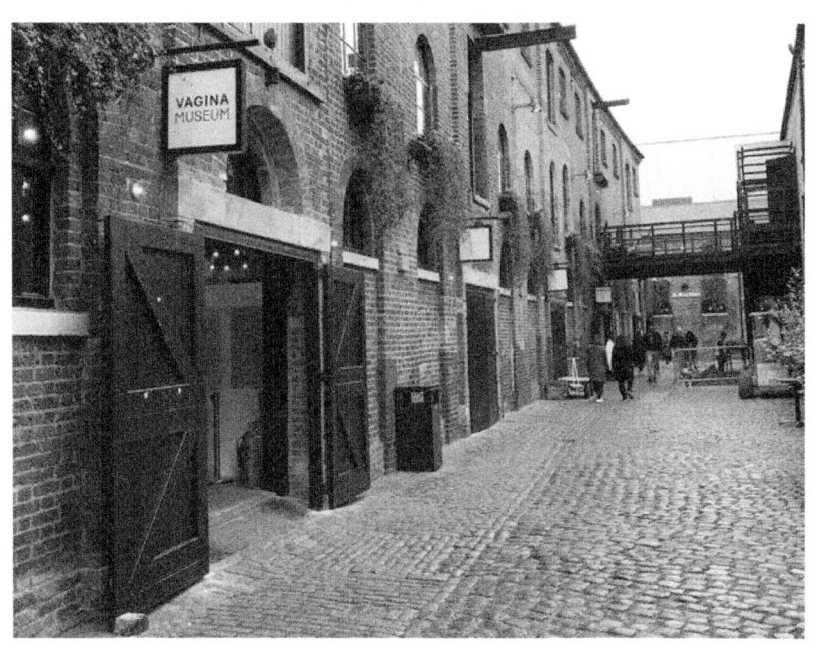

Vagina Museum entrance (Johnston, 2019).

Every woman's vagina is as unique as her fingerprint

and as unexplored as the depths of the ocean. For this reason, his approach deserves respect from any point of view.

The fact is *behind a happy woman is a happy vagina*.

Truths and preconceptions about the vagina that need to be told:

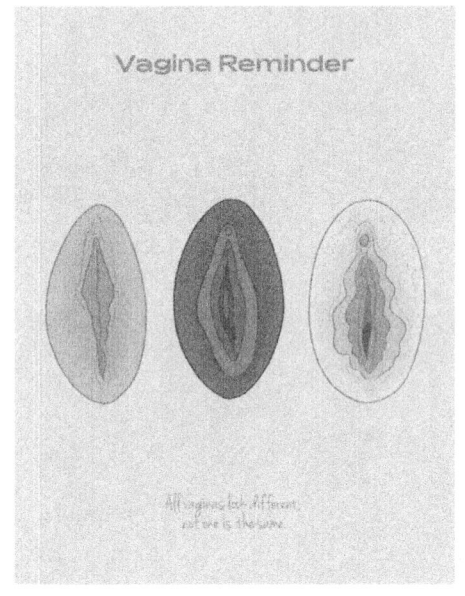

Vagina Reminder illustration by Charlotte Willcox (Gipson, 2020).

1. Vaginas exhibit diverse shapes and sizes, reflecting the natural variability inherent in every aspect of the human body.

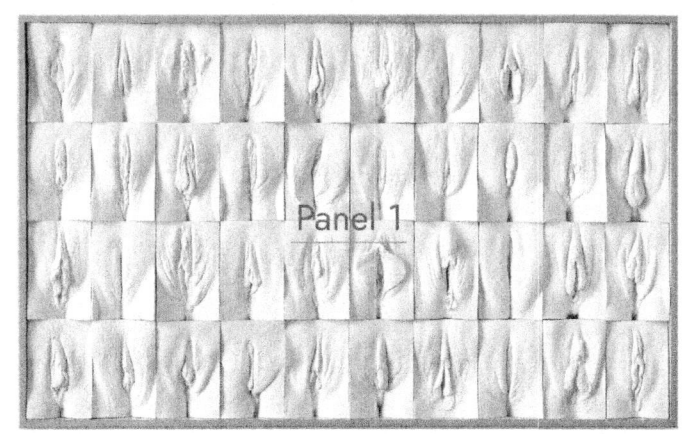

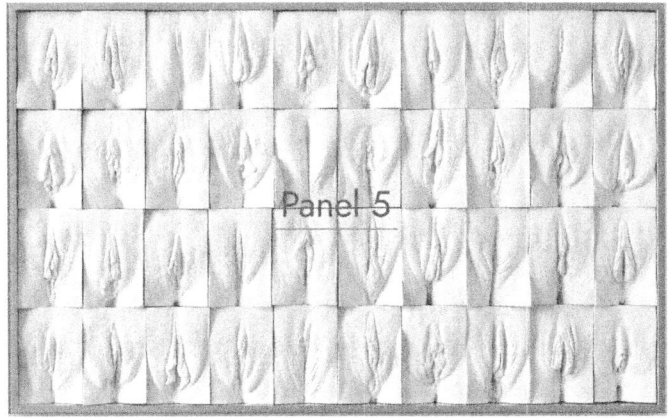

THE VAGINA CHRONICLES

Plaster casts of people's genitals (The great wall of vulva, 2024).

Plaster casts of people's genitals (The great wall of vulva, 2024).

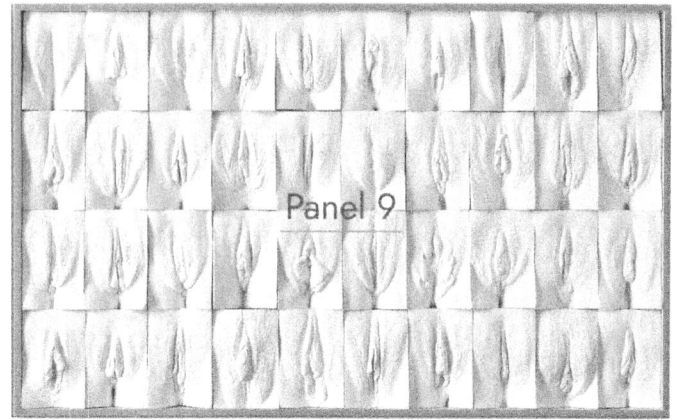

Plaster casts of people's genitals (The great wall of vulva, 2024).

2. Vaginas possess a self-cleaning mechanism: Maintaining a regulated PH balance and producing discharge are integral to the vagina's natural cleansing process, contributing to its overall health.
3. Vaginas undergoes significant transformations in the course of a woman's life: puberty, pregnancy, childbirth, and menopause represent stages marked by natural and normal changes.
4. Vaginal health prioritisation is crucial: Regular hygiene practices, such as gentle cleaning with water and mild soap, help prevent infections. It's advisable to avoid using fragranced soaps, bubble baths, or detergents.
5. Vaginal lubrication is a natural process: The vagina naturally produces lubrication to facilitate sexual activity. Factors like stress, medications, or hormonal changes can contribute to a lack of lubrication.

PREJUDICES AND MYTHS

Initiating discussions about vaginas requires a solid foundation built on respect, openness, and a committed effort to dispel myths. Gaining a clear understanding of the factual information related to vaginas plays a pivotal role in cultivating healthy attitudes and relationships. Now, let's explore some common prejudices and myths surrounding vaginas:

1. Vaginas are always clean and odourless: This misconception can lead to body shaming and unrealistic expectations. Vaginas have a natural odour and discharge that can vary from person to person and change depending on factors like the menstrual cycle, diet, and hygiene practices. It's important to understand that some level of odour and discharge is normal. The vagina should not smell like the Chelsea Flower Show.
2. Vaginas are meant to be tight: It's frequently misunderstood that a tight vagina signifies virginity or sexual purity. However, the reality is far more nuanced, the size and tightness of the vaginal canal differ among individuals and may evolve over time. This prevailing myth not only fosters unrealistic expectations but also contributes to the detrimental

practice of body shaming. It's crucial to dispel this misconception to foster a healthier understanding of women's bodies and promote positive attitudes towards sexuality.
3. Vaginas should be hairless: The idea that a hairless vagina is more attractive or hygienic is a common misconception. In reality, pubic hair serves the purpose of protecting the genital area, and it can be maintained or removed according to personal preference.
4. Vaginal appearance: The belief that vaginas should have a specific appearance or be symmetrical is another misconception. Vaginas come in various shapes, sizes, and colours, and there is no "normal" or one-size-fits-all standard for how they should look.

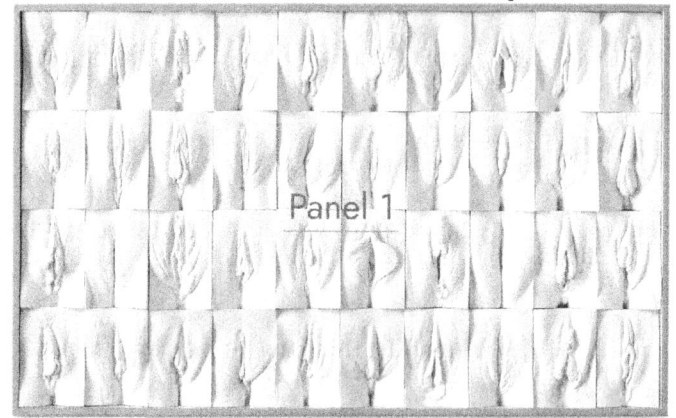

Plaster casts of people's genitals with different appearances (The great wall of vulva, 2024).

5. Vaginas are purely for sexual pleasure: While vaginas can provide sexual pleasure, they serve multiple functions, including menstruation, childbirth, and maintaining overall reproductive health.
6. The concept of "loose" or "stretched" vaginas: This notion often implies that frequent sexual activity or childbirth permanently stretches the vaginal canal.

In reality, the vagina is a muscular organ that can contract and expand, and it typically returns to its pre-sex or pre-pregnancy state.

7. The maintenance of vaginal health is crucial, considering the sensitivity of the area. Vaginas act as self-cleaning organs, and excessive cleansing or the application of harsh products may disrupt the delicate balance of the vaginal flora, potentially resulting in infections. Typically, a mild soap and water solution is adequate for gently cleaning the external genital area. It's essential to emphasise a balanced approach to promote optimal vaginal well-being.

8. Cotton underwear doesn't protect us more, so as feminist Canadian gynaecologist Dr Jen Gunter says, "If you hear the phrase, let the vagina breathe, laugh. Your vagina has no lungs. He doesn't want to get air, and he doesn't need oxygen. Sexy lace is a fine choice" (Gunter, 2019).

THE TOILET RULE

In an article by Dr Jen Gunter, a dynamic obstetrician and gynaecologist renowned for her work in women's health and advocacy for evidence-based information, the practice of front-to-back wiping for individuals with a vagina and anus is discussed as a longstanding hygiene principle. This ingrained guidance, passed down from early childhood through generations, serves to reduce the risk of bladder infections.

The rationale behind this wiping direction is primarily focused on preventing the transfer of faeces onto the skin, thereby avoiding introducing bacteria that can lead to urinary tract infections (UTIs). The concern is that these bacteria may settle in the vagina before ascending to the urethra and bladder.

It's crucial to note that after a bowel movement, faecal bacteria are already present on the skin from the toilet, and wiping with toilet paper alone may not completely remove them. The primary concern, especially for individuals beyond puberty, is to ensure that no faeces enter the vagina.

For those without medical conditions heightening this risk, the choice of how to wipe is largely at one's discretion, with a gentle approach recommended to prevent perianal skin irritation. In addition, a bidet is emphasised as a viable option. However, using wipes is cautioned against due to the potential for common irritation and even allergic reactions. The exception to this recommendation is for individuals with faecal incontinence who may need to clean on the go.

HAIR REMOVAL AND VAGINA

Hair removal for the pubic area offers various options, such as trimming, shaving, waxing or sugaring, laser hair removal, and depilatory creams. In the contemporary era, there is a widespread preoccupation with eliminating hair from all parts of the body, and the vagina has become a focal point in this pursuit. The methods employed to achieve the desired results vary, ranging from easy to fast, temporary to definitive, and inexpensive to costly, but they share a common element—PAIN.

The perplexity arises from the societal expectation that, unlike other mammals revelling in their fur, women should feel discomfort and embarrassment about their pubic hair. This expectation often leads to a sense of apology when facing oneself in the mirror. Choosing not to remove hair is not an admission of shame or a lack of commitment to self-improvement for attractiveness. It challenges the notion that a woman must conform to specific standards to be considered sexy.

The rituals of hair removal seem paradoxical—a voluntary journey to the metaphorical bed of torture where tears and screams accompany the quest for a "bald vagina" or stylised shapes such as heart-shaped or Brazilian. A contemporary variant, the "full-bush Brazilian," preserves the upper part of the vagina while completely depilating the rear area and lips. *Esthetician Jola Borzdynski said in an interview with New York Magazine that* the new trend is for those who feel a little hippy but have a weakness for kinky sex and that it is less painful than the standard Brazilian.

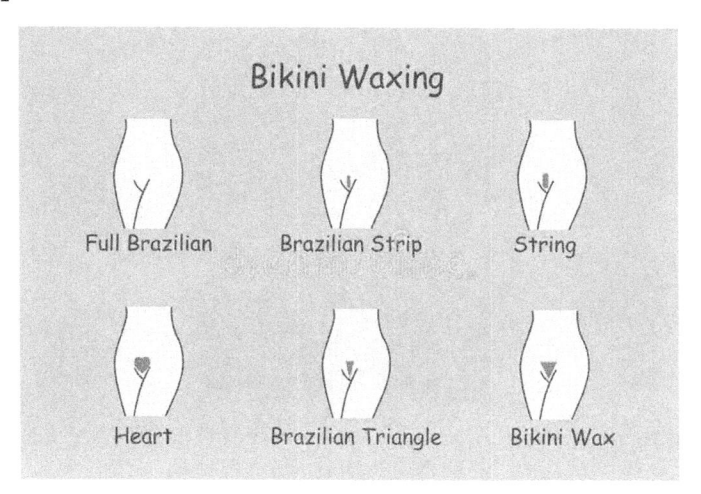

Hair removal styles (Cokal, 2018).

Some women assert that they undergo hair removal for hygiene reasons, but Dr Tami Rowen, a gynaecologist-obstetrician at the University of California in San Francisco, notes *"that hair growth serves a protective purpose for the sensitive genital tissues. Removing hair, particularly for women with heightened labial sensitivity, can increase the susceptibility to injuries, abrasions, abscesses, rashes, burns, or inflammation of hair follicles"*.

Choosing not to remove hair is not an admission of shame or a lack of commitment to self-improvement for attractiveness. It challenges the notion that a woman must conform to specific standards to be considered sexy.

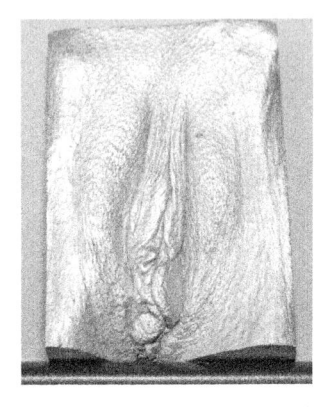

Sculpture of the genital area without hair (Saatchi Art, 2022).

In conclusion, the decision to engage in partial or total hair removal of the vagina is a personal choice for each woman. What is crucial is recognising that the natural presence of pubic hair is normal, and no woman should feel the need to apologise for it.

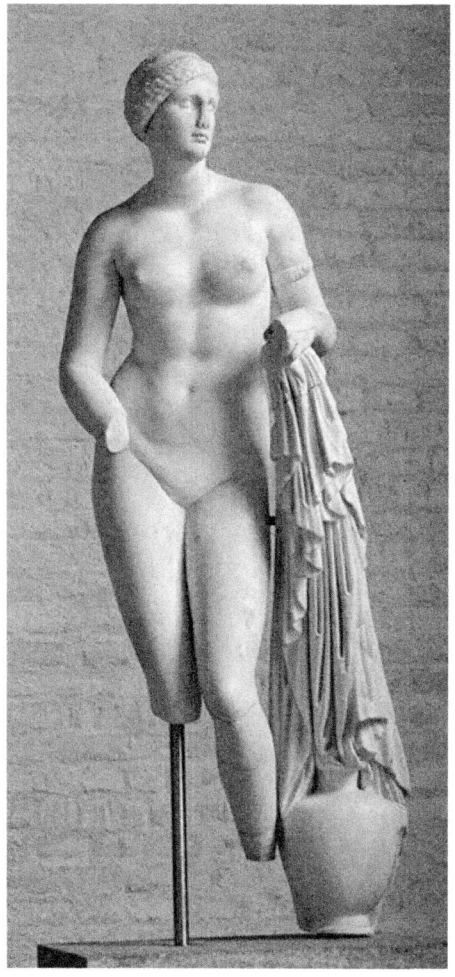

Sculpture showing lack of vaginal hair (Gipson, 2020).

MENSTRUATION AND PERIOD-POVERTY

Menstruation or period is a completely normal process that occurs in girls between the ages of ten and sixteen. In contrast, the average age of onset is twelve years. At this point, I would like to say that I do not intend to refer to facts related to medical science since I neither have the special knowledge nor the intention. I would prefer to cite some social issues connected to the period process, the parameters of which plague modern Western societies as well.

This is the so-called Period Poverty.

Breaking the Chains of Period Poverty: A Call for Equality

Period poverty is a serious worldwide problem that affects millions of people, mostly women and girls, who cannot afford to use adequate sanitation facilities and menstrual hygiene products. This problem transcends borders, income levels, and cultures, impacting the dignity, health, and opportunities of those who experience it.

Understanding Period Poverty

Period poverty is a multifaceted issue that encompasses various challenges:

1. **Inadequate Access to Menstrual Products:** Many individuals cannot access or afford menstrual products such as pads, tampons, or menstrual cups. This lack of access can lead to the use of improvised, unhygienic alternatives like rags or paper.
2. **Poor Sanitation and Hygiene Facilities:** Period poverty can be made worse by inadequate sanitary facilities in public areas, workplaces, and schools. Lack of access to hygienic, private restrooms with running water and suitable disposal methods may deter people from managing their periods in an efficient manner.
3. **Stigma and Shame:** The cultural stigma surrounding menstruation can lead to embarrassment and secrecy, making it difficult for individuals to discuss their needs openly, seek support, or advocate for change.

Consequences of Period Poverty

Period poverty has far-reaching consequences on individuals and society as a whole:

1. **Health Implications:** Using unhygienic materials can lead to infections, urinary tract issues, and other health problems during menstruation. Period poverty causes stress and anxiety, which can exacerbate mental health issues.
2. **Education and Employment:** For many, period poverty can lead to absenteeism from school

and work, hindering their education and career opportunities. Girls missing school due to menstruation may fall behind in their studies, perpetuating gender disparities.
3. **Gender Inequality:** Period poverty perpetuates stereotypes and marginalises women and girls because it is intrinsically linked to gender inequality. This restriction limits their potential and feeds the poverty cycle.

Addressing Period Poverty

To combat period poverty, we need a multi-faceted approach that includes the following:

1. **Accessible and Affordable Menstrual Products:** Governments, NGOs, and private enterprises should work together to ensure that menstrual products are widely available and affordable. Subsidies, tax exemptions, and donation programs can help make these products more accessible.
2. **Education and Awareness:** Comprehensive menstrual education programs should be integrated into school curricula to reduce stigma and empower individuals to confidently manage their periods. This should include information on reusable and sustainable options like menstrual cups.
3. **Improved Sanitation Facilities:** Investment in clean, private restrooms in schools, workplaces, and public spaces is crucial. These facilities should have water, proper disposal methods, and hygiene supplies.
4. **Community Initiatives:** Breaking the taboo around menstruation is largely the responsibility of grassroots organisations and local authorities.

Workshops, advocacy campaigns, and support groups can reduce stigma and promote significant change.

Period poverty is not just a matter of lacking access to menstrual products; it is an issue that permeates every aspect of an individual's life, from their health and education to their self-esteem and opportunities. Achieving menstrual equity is a matter of social justice and a crucial step towards gender equality and a more inclusive society. By comprehensively addressing period poverty through accessible products, education, and improved sanitation, we can help break the chains that have bound too many for too long. It's time to normalise menstruation, raise our voices, and make the world a place where no one has to suffer the indignity of period poverty.

The example of Scotland

Scotland has made great progress in tackling the problem of period poverty, which is the inability to purchase menstrual hygiene products because of financial limitations. Here's an overview of how Scotland has addressed this issue:

1. Free Period Products in Schools: In 2018, Scotland became the first country to provide free menstrual products in all schools, colleges, and universities. This initiative aimed to ensure that students would not miss out on their education due to a lack of access to period products.

2. The Period Products (Free Provision) (Scotland) Act 2021: In November 2020, the Scottish Parliament unanimously passed the Period Products (Free Provision) (Scotland) Act. Scotland has made great progress in tackling the problem of period poverty, which is the inability to purchase menstrual hygiene products because of financial limitations.
3. Access to Products in Public Places: The Act goes beyond educational institutions and public buildings, as it also requires public bodies to make period products available in other community settings where they may be needed.
4. Creation of a Menstrual Products Taskforce: The Menstrual Products Taskforce was established by the Scottish government to supervise the Act's implementation and guarantee accessibility. The taskforce has been assigned the responsibility of offering direction and overseeing the delivery of period products.
5. Raising Awareness: Scotland has also worked to reduce the stigma surrounding menstruation and period poverty through public awareness campaigns. By openly discussing the issue, they aim to reduce the shame associated with menstruation and encourage open conversations.
6. Expanding the Initiative: Besides schools and public buildings, efforts are ongoing to ensure that period products are readily available in various settings, including workplaces, public transportation, and other locations where people may require them.

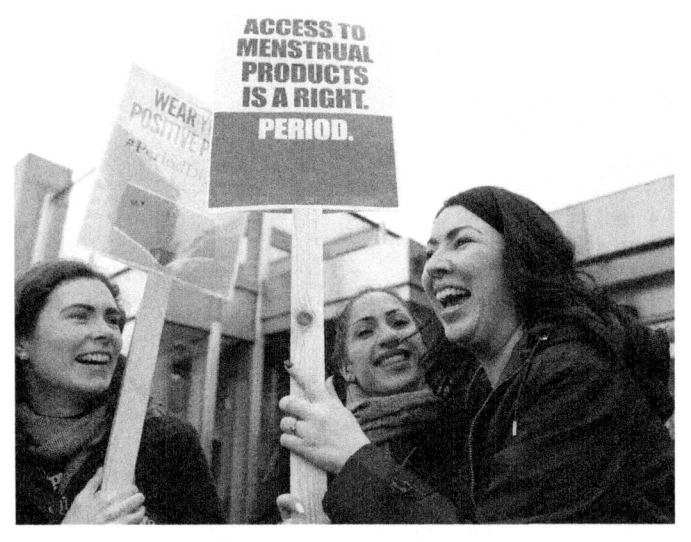

Scottish campaign (Wamsley, 2020).

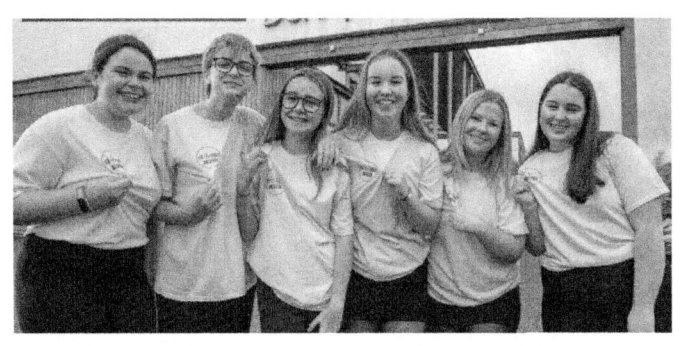

Denny High School in Scotland campaign (Connor, 2022).

These measures represent a comprehensive approach to tackling period poverty in Scotland by providing free access to period products in various public places and institutions and promoting open dialogue about menstruation. Other countries and regions have also been inspired by Scotland's approach and have begun implementing similar initiatives to address period poverty.

MENOPAUSE

Just as the onset of menstruation holds significance in a woman's life, so does its cessation. In recent years, there has been a growing discourse surrounding menopause, encompassing discussions about its symptoms, treatments, and the societal implications it carries. Many women find it challenging to embrace the changes associated with menopause, affecting both their physical well-being and mental health.

To confront this transformative phase, often referred to as "the beast," an increasing number of women turn to nutritional supplements, hormone treatments, and various medical interventions. The psychosomatic cost of menopause is often overlooked, even though experts present it as an inevitable life stage linked to psychological, sexual, and physical liberation. There is a common misconception that many women are unable to understand its intricacies, leaving them unprepared for the emotional obstacles that could occur.

Dr. Gunter succinctly captures the essence of menopause, describing it as *puberty in reverse.* Menopause is a natural biological process signifying the conclusion of a woman's reproductive years. Typically occurring in the late 40s or early 50s, the age of onset varies among women. It is officially defined as the point when a woman has not had a menstrual period for 12 consecutive months.

During menopause, the ovaries gradually reduce the production of hormones, such as estrogen and progesterone, which regulate the menstrual cycle and fertility. This hormonal shift leads to a range of physical and emotional symptoms, including:

1. Irregular menstrual periods: In the years leading up to menopause (perimenopause), women may experience changes in their menstrual cycles, including irregular periods.
2. Hot flashes: Sudden feelings of heat that can cause sweating and reddening skin, often accompanied by rapid heartbeat.
3. Night sweats: Hot flashes that occur at night, leading to sweating and discomfort.
4. Vaginal dryness: A decrease in estrogen levels can result in vaginal dryness, which can lead to discomfort during sexual intercourse. Don't use fragranced products or wipes because they increase irritation, but do moisturise with coconut oil or unfragranced petroleum jelly.

5. Mood swings: Hormonal changes can affect mood and may lead to irritability, anxiety, and mood swings.
6. Sleep disturbances: Many women experience difficulty sleeping or insomnia during menopause.
7. Changes in libido: Some women may experience a decrease in sexual desire during menopause.
8. Weight gain: Changes in metabolism and hormonal fluctuations can lead to weight gain, particularly around the abdomen.
9. Osteoporosis: The loss of estrogen can decrease bone density, increasing the risk of osteoporosis.
10. Changes in hair and skin: Some women may notice changes in their hair and skin texture due to hormonal shifts.

It's important to note that not all women experience the same symptoms during menopause, and the severity and duration of these symptoms can vary widely. While menopause is a natural part of the ageing process, healthcare providers can offer guidance and treatments to help manage and alleviate some of the symptoms, such as hormone replacement therapy, lifestyle changes, and medications.

Menopause does mark the end of a woman's fertility, but it can also bring a sense of freedom from menstruation and birth control concerns for many women. It's a transitional phase in a woman's life that should be understood and managed to promote overall well-being and health.

But apart from the symptoms I mentioned above, Menopause is a major life transition that affects not only physical health but also emotional well-being and social interactions. As such, it presents women with a variety of social and psychological challenges. Here are some of the social problems that women may encounter during menopause:

1. Stigmatisation and Misunderstanding: Menopause is sometimes stigmatised, and there is a lack of knowledge and compassion about the mental and physical changes that women go through. This may contribute to societal prejudices and unfavourable preconceptions about menopausal women.
2. Workplace Issues: Women going through menopause may face challenges at work due to symptoms such as hot flashes, mood swings, and fatigue. These symptoms can affect productivity and job performance, and some women may find it difficult to discuss their needs with employers or colleagues.
3. Relationship Strain: Menopausal symptoms like mood swings, irritability, and changes in libido can strain intimate relationships. Communication and understanding between partners are crucial during this time to maintain a healthy and supportive relationship.
4. Body Image Concerns: Menopause can bring about changes in weight and body shape. Some women may experience a decline in self-esteem and body image issues, which can impact their social lives and confidence.
5. Social Isolation: Menopausal symptoms, including

sleep disturbances and mood swings, can lead to social withdrawal. Women may avoid social activities or gatherings due to discomfort or fatigue, which can result in isolation and loneliness.
6. Lack of Support: A lack of social and emotional support can exacerbate menopausal symptoms. Friends, family, and healthcare providers should provide understanding, encouragement, and information to help women navigate this transition.
7. Impact on Social Activities: Menopause symptoms such as weariness and night sweats can interfere with routine social interactions, making women turn down invitations or skip social gatherings.
8. Mental Health Challenges: Some women experience depression, anxiety, or mood disorders during menopause, which can further impact their social relationships and interactions.

Suppose you add up all of the above. In that case, you will understand that the burden that accumulates on women's shoulders during the menopause period is heavy and multidimensional. So perhaps we can understand why more and more women these days resort to menopause centres, where by following holistic methods and metabolic health programs, they try to support themselves psychosomatically.

According to the Global Wellness Summit, the menopause market will be worth $600 billion by 2025, with more than 1 billion women reaching menopause by then. It is really important for women to include health issues in their agenda.

SENSITIVE AREA AND EXERCISE

The exercise of the sensitive area that not only improves sex but also prevents unwanted incontinence is called *Kegel*.

Engaging in pelvic floor muscle exercises, commonly referred to as Kegel exercises, proves to be an effective method for fortifying the muscles in the pelvic area, particularly those surrounding the vagina. Strengthening these pelvic floor muscles can improve bladder control, increase sexual satisfaction, and promote overall pelvic health. The following outlines the steps for performing Kegel exercises:

1. **Find Your Pelvic Floor Muscles:** The first step is identifying the pelvic floor muscles. You can do this by stopping the flow of urine midstream or imagining you're trying to prevent passing gas. The muscles you use for these actions are your pelvic floor muscles.
2. **Get in the Right Position:** You can perform Kegel exercises in any position, but it's often easiest to start seated or lying down. Make sure your muscles are relaxed.

3. **Perform the Exercise:** Squeeze your pelvic floor muscles for a count of 3-5 seconds, then release for the same amount of time. Gradually work your way up to longer squeezes and releases. Aim for 10-15 repetitions in a single set.
4. **Maintain Your Breathing:** Keep breathing normally while doing the exercises. Avoid holding your breath.
5. **Don't Overdo It:** Start with a comfortable number of repetitions and progressively increase them over time to avoid overstretching these muscles. Excessive Kegel exercises can wear out your muscles.
6. **Consistency is Key:** To see improvements in pelvic muscle strength, consistency is important. Aim to do Kegel exercises daily or as advised by your healthcare provider.
7. **Progressive Exercises:** As your pelvic floor muscles get stronger, you can increase the intensity by squeezing harder or holding the contraction longer.

You can engage in Kegel exercises at home without any specialised equipment or in a gym setting, as they do not necessitate special machinery or weights. The crucial aspect is to execute these exercises accurately and regularly.

If you're uncertain about the proper execution of Kegel exercises or harbour concerns regarding your pelvic health, seeking advice from a healthcare professional is advisable. A gynaecologist or a pelvic health physical therapist can offer guidance, assess your technique, and may propose customised exercises or techniques based on your individual requirements.

Dr Arnold Kegel was an American gynaecologist who is best known for developing a set of exercises now commonly referred to as "Kegel exercises." Kegel exercises, which target issues like urinary incontinence, pelvic organ prolapse, and sexual function, are frequently recommended for both men and women. They are designed to strengthen the pelvic floor muscles that support the bladder, uterus, and sexual function.

Dr Kegel's work in this area, particularly in the 1940s, helped raise awareness about the importance of pelvic floor health. The exercises he developed involve contracting and relaxing the pelvic floor muscles, and they are often taught to individuals by healthcare professionals to improve their pelvic muscle strength and control. These exercises can be beneficial for various health conditions, including those related to childbirth, ageing, and certain medical procedures.

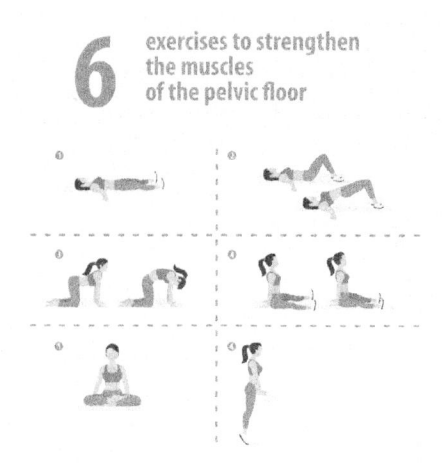

Pelvic floor strengthening exercises (Centerforurologiccare.com)

VULVOPLASTY

Vulvoplasty is a surgical procedure that involves the reconstruction or alteration of the vulva, which is the external genitalia in females. It is typically performed for various medical and cosmetic reasons, and the specific goals and techniques can vary depending on the individual's needs. Here are some key points about vulvoplasty:

1. Medical Indications:
   - Congenital conditions: Vulvoplasty may be performed to address congenital abnormalities or intersex variations of the vulva.
   - Trauma or injury: Some individuals may require vulvoplasty after an accident or injury that affects the vulva.
   - Gender-affirming surgery: Vulvoplasty is often a component of gender-confirmation surgery (also known as gender reassignment surgery) for transgender women.
2. Goals of Vulvoplasty:
   - Reconstruction: In cases of congenital abnormalities or trauma, the primary goal is to create a functional and aesthetically pleasing vulva.
   - Gender confirmation: In gender-affirming surgery, the aim is to create female external genitalia that align with the patient's gender identity.

3. Techniques:
- The specific technique used in vulvoplasty can vary widely depending on the patient's needs and the surgeon's expertise. Common procedures may include labiaplasty (surgery to alter the labia minora or majora), clitoroplasty (surgery to create or modify the clitoris), and vaginoplasty (surgery to create or modify the vaginal canal).
- The surgical approach may be informed by the patient's desired outcomes, the surgeon's experience, and tissue availability for reconstruction.

4. Risks and Complications:
- As with any surgical procedure, vulvoplasty carries potential risks and complications, including infection, scarring, changes in sensation, and unsatisfactory aesthetic results. Discussing these risks with a qualified surgeon before undergoing the procedure is important.

5. Recovery:
- The length of the procedure determines how long it takes to recover from vulvoplasty. It is possible for patients to experience pain, bruising, and swelling; full recovery could take several weeks to months.
- Post-operative care and follow-up visits with the surgeon are essential to monitor the healing process and address any issues that may arise.

Vulvoplasty is a highly specialised surgical procedure. If someone is thinking about it, they should speak with skilled surgeons who specialise in the field, whether for health reasons or to promote gender identity. Additionally, patients should be well-informed about the procedure, the expected outcomes, and potential risks before deciding.

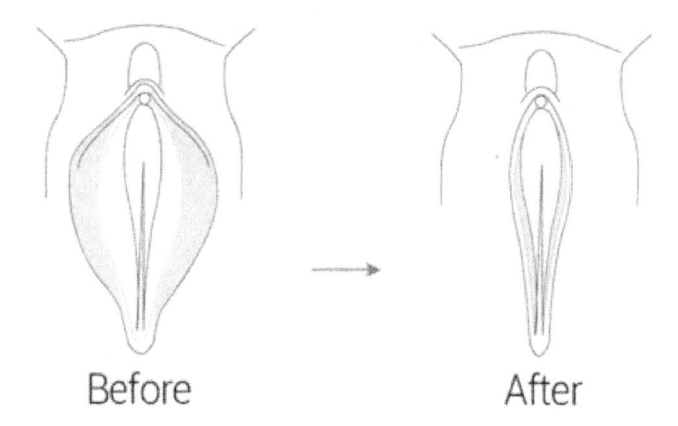

Before → After

Illustration of before and after vulvoplasty (Quartz Clinique, 2023).

VAGINAL BLEACHING

Vaginal bleaching is a cosmetic procedure that involves lightening the skin around the vaginal area to achieve a more uniform or lighter skin tone. The practice of vaginal bleaching is primarily driven by cosmetic and aesthetic concerns and is not without potential risks.

Here are some key points to consider about vaginal bleaching:

~ Lack of Medical Necessity: Vaginal bleaching is not medically necessary and is purely a cosmetic procedure. It is not endorsed by medical professionals or regulatory agencies.

~ Safety Concerns: There are possible hazards associated with using vaginal bleaching products and methods. Certain products might have harsh chemicals in them, which could cause allergic reactions, skin irritation, or harm to the delicate skin around the genitalia.

~ Lack of Regulation: Many products used for vaginal bleaching are not regulated or approved by health authorities.

This means there is limited oversight, and the safety and effectiveness of these products can be questionable.

~ Alternatives: If someone is concerned about thappearance of their genital area, there are safer and less invasive alternatives, such as consulting a dermatologist for advice on skin-lightening options, if desired. It's essential to prioritise one's safety and health.

~ Psychological and Societal Factors: The desire for vaginal bleaching can be influenced by societal beauty standards and personal body image concerns. It's essential to consider the psychological and emotional aspects of this choice.

~ Consult a Professional: If someone is determined to explore vaginal bleaching, they should consult a qualified healthcare professional or dermatologist who can provide guidance and, if necessary, recommend safe and appropriate treatments.

~ Self-Acceptance: Ultimately, the most important aspects of one's body are self-acceptance and self-esteem. It's important to remember that natural skin tone and appearance variations are entirely normal and should be celebrated.

In conclusion, vaginal bleaching is a cosmetic procedure that carries potential risks. Anyone considering such a procedure should consult with a healthcare professional and carefully consider the reasons behind their decision, keeping in mind the importance of self-acceptance and overall well-being.

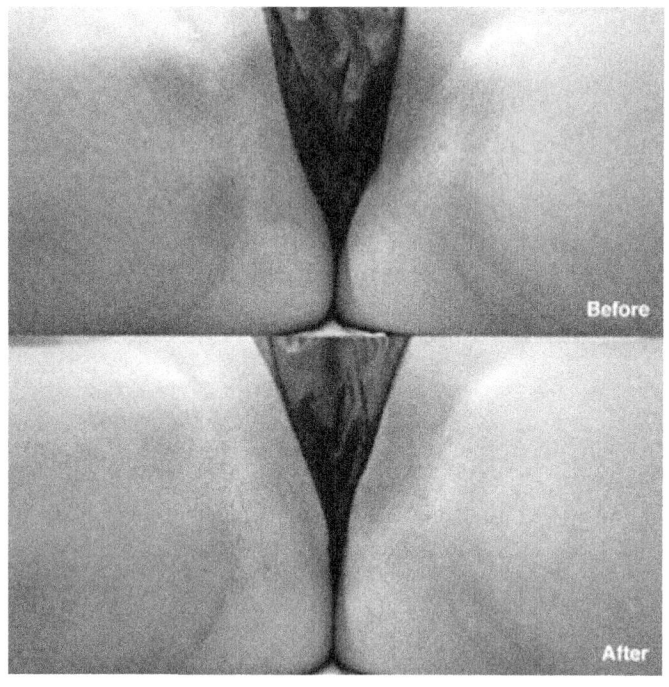

Vaginal bleaching photos before and after (Real Styling Solutions, 2022).

CONTROVERSIAL VAGINAL CARE RECOMMENDATIONS

Put stone "eggs" inside your vagina: the strictly guarded secret of Chinese royalty in antiquity, queens and concubines used them to stay in shape for emperors, Jade Egg brings increased sexual energy and pleasure.

Steam your vagina: The idea behind vaginal steaming is to use steam to cleanse and revitalise the vagina.

Pineapple juice makes your vagina smell better, or using sugar down there to make it "sticky" and "sweet", or decorating your vagina "it's like having a sparkly secret in your pants".

These are some suggestions that celebrities have occasionally offered over time. It's advisable to dismiss these recommendations, as they either involve pseudoscientific and potentially harmful practices or are mere misconceptions that could potentially lead to vaginal infections.

PART TWO

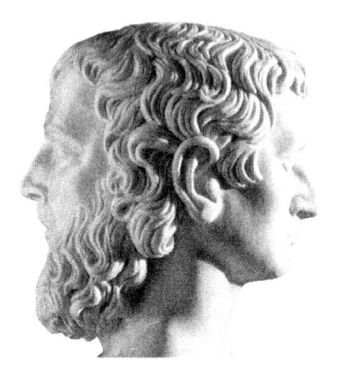

A statue of the Roman god Janus (Wayne, 2013).

Before starting the second part of the book,, I would like to refer to a mythical person, Janus, and explain why.

Janus was one of the most important deities of the ancient Romans and was depicted with two faces. One was bearded, aged and symbolised the past, while the other was clean-shaven, youthful and symbolised the future. This counterpoint symbolised change and transitions, such as progress from the past to the future, from one state to another, from one vision to another, and the growth of young people into adulthood. Janus represented time in a way, since he could see into the past with one face and into the future with the other.

This is how I would like to approach both the issue of Female Genital Mutilation (FGM) and the issue of Menstrual Ostracism.

These two practices, the first involving mutilation and the second ostracising women, target the essence of female nature. Despite their roots dating back hundreds of years, they continue to thrive today.

Thus, I will not only focus on the analytical presentation of data related to these issues, seeing them as events related to the past, but I will also refer to the optimistic struggles aimed at eliminating these practices from the world map in the future.

FEMALE GENITAL MUTILATION

Esther Lankeu, a Kenyan survivor and anti-FGM activist: "As a survivor of FGM who has lived with the consequences of the cut, I will not allow my daughters to go through it and will keep using my experiences to advocate against this practice."

Maryum Saifee, an FGM survivor and activist in the United States: "FGM destroys the childhoods of girls and women. We need to end FGM so girls can live in dignity, free from violence, and realise their full potential.

"Speak up! Even if you are not directly affected, it is important we create a world where everyone has zero tolerance for FGM."

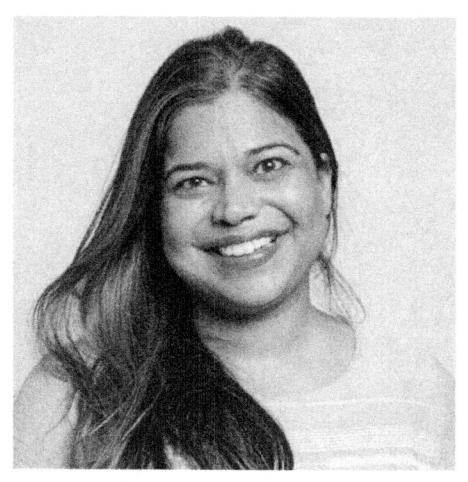

Photo of Maryum Saifee (Kearl, 2021).

Damaris is from Kenya. She underwent FGM at age 11. At the time, she had no idea what it really was.

"I didn't know where I was going to be cut. I wanted to run, but they held me back. I was crying so much."

Afterwards, Damaris was forced to marry. As a result of FGM, having sex and giving birth to her baby was agonising.

Luckily, she heard of ActionAid's women's group. Damaris says the group has made a huge difference in her life - she now feels safe and supported, and is learning practical skills to help her in the future.

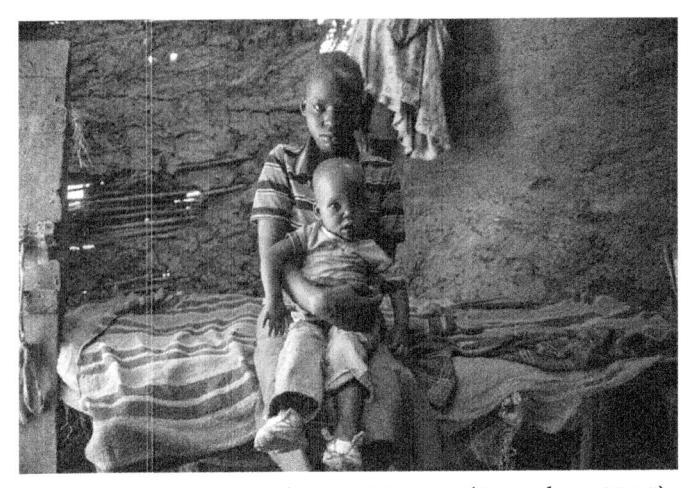

Damaris with her daughter at 14 years (Waterlow, 2015).

"Thanks to the group, I feel better daily," she says. "We talk about our life experiences. I tell them how bad and sad it feels to be married off to someone you do not know. After talking to the group and letting everything go out of my head, I feel at peace with myself.

"We also learn business skills. I'd like a shop where I could sell maize flour, sugar, batteries and many more things. ActionAid gives us hope and strength. Every time I leave the meetings, I feel really hopeful."

Istar's Story:

"My name is Istar. I am 28 years old mother and a student. I would like to share my experience of undergoing FGM. This will be the first time I've ever written about my experience. This will be the one chance the child within my voice will be heard. I was 6 years old when it happened, all I know is that I was playing outside our house with other children who lived nearby, I also remember a lot of relatives and family friends where at the house, a lot of food and sweets were cooked that day, but strangely my parents weren't there, didn't think much of it at the time.

The nightmare started as my younger sister was called into the house by aunts I followed but was told to wait outside again. I didn't think much of it then. One of my neighbour daughter, who was playing with us, came to me, "You must be excited." My response, "What for?" I didn't know what she was talking about. "You will be a big girl now; all you have to do is be very brave and don't cry". I still didn't understand what she meant. When she explained what was going to happen to me, all I wanted was for my mom to come and rescue me, I ran so fast, trying to hide in the house at the same time I could hear my little sister scream, I had never heard such scream, even today when I shut my eyes I can hear her screaming".

"Get Istar; it's her turn", I could hear my aunt saying. I kept running around the house until I got caught and dragged to the table where I was surrounded by two of my aunts, one of our neighbours and two men. I didn't know who they were at the time but realised that one of them was the circumcisers well that's what people call them if I had given them a title it would be the children's butcher".

"The other man grabbed hold of my legs, trying to pull them apart; I fought him as much as I could, but I was only six years old, and I had no energy left within me when he succeeded, I remember him saying to me, "Behave you silly girl and stop crying it doesn't hurt". My lower part of my body was out of my control I tried to move my upper part of my body, but my aunts held me down and stuffed big cloth in my mouth so I wouldn't scream so loud, god that was all they were worried about. As this was happening, all I wanted was my mother. She was always there for me; WHY NOT THIS TIME"?

"When he was done, I felt so ashamed that these people saw my private parts, and these men actually touched it and hurt me. Brave girl Istar, everybody said. I remember getting a lot of sweets, toys and money to congratulate me. At the time, I thought you were part of these people now, and you are treated differently. "The very special girl now". Again, as this was happening to me, all I wanted was my mommy".

"As I got older, I realised the damage FGM has caused me physically and mentally. I was led to believe I had type1 but later, in my early twenties, I realised I've actually undergone Type2, but the mental scar I carry today is tough to explain I've blocked it out for many years pretended that it never happened but I could no longer ignore it especially after my beautiful little girl was born, I knew as a mother I couldn't let that happened to my daughter but that meant facing the demons from the past".

Aisha- from Singapore:

"I was told as a child that every girl had to go through it. There is basically nobody that you know who hasn't gone through it. I believed everything my mother said. I had an inter-racial Muslim marriage. I realised my sexual desire plummeted, and I wasn't really interested in sex much longer. In a private conversation with my husband, I learned that Female Genital Cutting (FGC) is practiced in many Asian countries. Surprisingly, as a Muslim in his own country, FGC is not a common practice. In his country, none of his sisters underwent FGC. I had my daughter at home, assisted by my husband. The natural delivery left a stinging, burning sensation on my clitoris region. I thought it would disappear, but it lasted much longer than expected.

A few months passed, and I still felt a strange sensation

in my clitoris region. When I urinated, it felt like someone had punched me – it was sore. I refused to go for a health check-up as I didn't want anyone to touch me. I didn't want to feel it myself.

It has been almost 10 months since my baby's birth, and my husband and I have not resumed intimacy. Initially, I feared potential pain. Subsequently, I wanted to avoid the intermittent sore sensation in my clitoris region. Thirdly, my sexual drive or desire was low, primarily due to breastfeeding.

I deeply pondered: Why am I still feeling this? Why does it still feel sore? Is it because of the FGC that my mother made sure I underwent when I was still a baby? I had my daughter at home, assisted by my husband. The natural delivery left a stinging, burning sensation on my clitoris region. I thought it would disappear, but it lasted much longer than expected.

In 2016, at 30 years of age, it affected me. I was upset that my mother did it purely due to social pressure. Even if you're an educated woman, social pressure can still influence how you decide. I was in a mosque a few weeks back, and a lady in her 50-60s approached me and chatted about my baby. She handed me her name card, which indicated her business services. It read, "sunat perempuan". I was shocked and disappointed. This is being done by an unlicensed passerby who easily roamed the community promoting her services" (Equality Now, 2020). (all the above experiences are from the page of Equality Now, which is an international organisation that advocates for a world where women and girls have control over their bodies).

But what exactly is Genital Female Mutilation (GFM)?

Female genital mutilation (FGM), or female circumcision (FC), or female genital cutting (FGC), or gudnin, is a traditional social practice of cutting parts of the external genitalia of girls and young women to uphold a cultural practice of a rite of passage to womanhood and to curb sexuality. It is classified by the World Health Organization (WHO) into four major types.

Type 1 FGM

Clitoridectomy: partial or total removal of the clitoris (a small, sensitive and erectile part of the female genitals) and, in very rare cases, only the prepuce (the fold of skin surrounding the clitoris).

This practice is extremely painful and distressing, damages sexually sensitive skin and is an infection risk.

Type 2 FGM

Excision: partial or total removal of the clitoris and the labia minora, with or without excision of the labia majora (the labia are the 'lips' that surround the vagina).

This practice is extremely painful and distressing, damages sexually sensitive skin and is an infection risk.

Type 3 FGM

Infibulation: narrowing of the vaginal opening through the creation of a covering seal. The seal is formed by cutting and sewing over the outer labia, with or without removal of the clitoris or inner labia.

This practice is extremely painful and distressing, damages sexually sensitive skin and is an on-going infection risk. The closing over of the vagina and the urethra leaves women with a very small opening in which to pass urine and menstrual fluid. The opening can be so small that it needs to be cut open to be able to have sexual intercourse. Cutting is also needed to give birth and can cause complications which harm both mother and baby.

Type 4 FGM

Other: all other harmful procedures to the female genitalia for non-medical purposes, e.g. pricking, piercing, incising, scraping, stretching and cauterising the genital area.

In some communities, after the torturous process, the girl's legs are tied together to immobilise them for 10 to 14 days to close the wound.

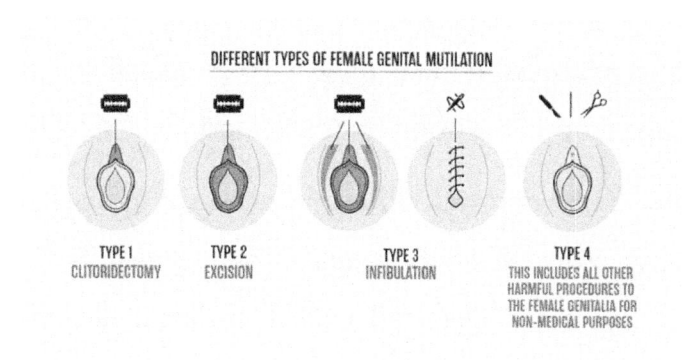

Types of FGM (Varma, 2023).

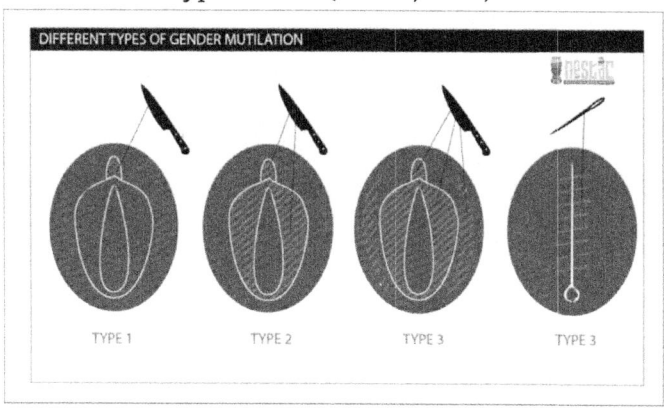

Types of FGM (The Live Life, 2021).

It's important to grasp that FGM is not inherently tied to any specific religion; rather, it is a cultural and social custom prevalent in certain regions with diverse religious backgrounds. FGM is practised in various Christian, Muslim, and indigenous religious communities, as well as in non-religious contexts. It is imperative to recognise that the major world religions do not condone the practice of FGM and that religious texts do not expressly command it. The main causes of FGM are social and cultural practices that are strongly rooted in customs and ideas related to femininity, purity, and the passage from childhood to adulthood.

While some communities may attempt to justify FGM by referencing cultural or religious norms, these justifications are not universally accepted within religious communities. However, it is observed that FGM occurs with the tacit tolerance of religions, governments, and even social scientists.

The young girls are uninformed about the procedure ahead of time. On the contrary, they anticipate a familial celebration filled with gifts and joy. The operation is conducted by an often older woman possessing healing knowledge, esteemed within the local community. The tools employed are rudimentary and rarely sanitised—rusty razors or knives, broken glass, stones, fingernails, and whatever is deemed suitable for the occasion.

The venue for this "operation" is typically a hut

situated away from the settlement, ensuring the girl's cries go unheard, preventing panic among other girls in the community. Until her wounds heal, the girl stays in this remote hut; only then is she considered "clean" enough to be allowed back into the community.

The girl's return hinges on the outcome of the "operation," and due to the absence of sanitary precautions, numerous girls frequently succumb to either bleeding or fatal infections. Girls subjected to FGM can range in age from 0 to 12, with instances of older women also undergoing FGM.

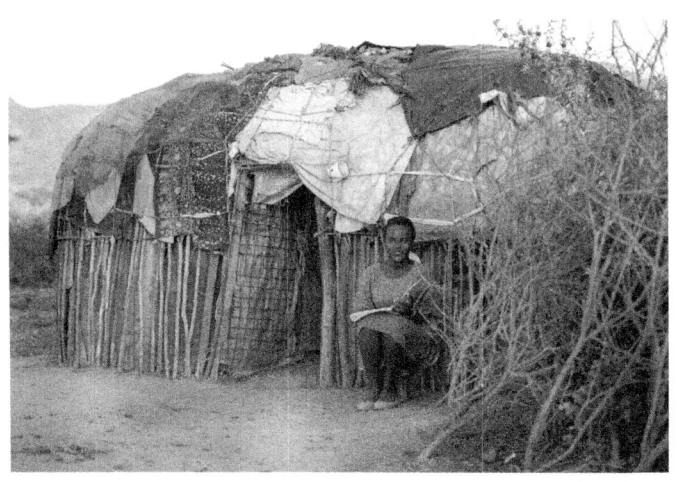

Typical rural homes where FGM in is mainly practised (USAID, 2021).

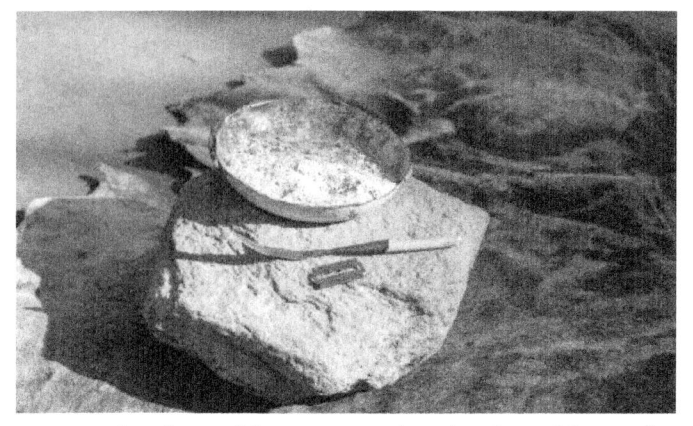

Types of tools used in FGM practices (Action Aid, 2016).

The worldwide scientific community and activist organisations vehemently condemn a cultural practice that amounts to a violation of female nature—a crime seeking to subjugate women through physical punishment. This ongoing suffering turns into a lifetime burden for women and is a type of gender-based violence intended to give men control over femininity. Men are the main winners because they want to maintain a woman's virginity, make sure she stays faithful after marriage, and indulge in their own sexual desires.

In fact, it is a toxic culture which, as the broadcaster, activist and author Thom Hartmann asserts, "Culture can be healthy or toxic, nurturing or murderous" (Thom Hartmann, The Last Hours of Ancient Sunlight: The Fate of the World and What We Can Do About It Before It's Too Late NY: Three Rivers

Press, But we would say that it takes place under the tacit tolerance of religions, states, and even social scientists 2000, 164).

The reasons for FGM are complex and can vary across different communities and individuals, but they generally fall into the following categories:

1. Cultural and Tradition: FGM is often deeply rooted in cultural traditions and is considered a rite of passage or a way to mark a girl's transition to womanhood. But this transition is torturous, and the person goes through pain of soul and body from innocence to maturity. FGM-practicing communities might see it as a vital component of their cultural identity. It can be difficult to stop FGM because many communities see it as a custom that was carried down from their forefathers. There's often strong pressure to conform to the customs of their forebears.

   Elders and traditional birth attendants play a crucial role in perpetuating FGM. They are the custodians of these traditions and are responsible for carrying out the procedure. The authority of these individuals is highly respected and rarely questioned.

2. Social Pressure and Acceptance: In some communities, not conforming to the practice of FGM can result in social ostracism or stigmatisation. Women and girls may undergo FGM to gain social acceptance and access to marriage

opportunities. Individual freedom is subordinated to the collective. This is what social scientists call "integration anxiety". Any differentiation from the social group leads to social deviation of the individual, who now loses his social identity and status. Whereas FGM gives women something like their coveted "entry card" into social becoming. In communities where all women have FGM and all girls are expected to have it, FGM can seem normal. It can seem like there is no other choice, and it is very difficult for girls to challenge these traditions. Women who resist or speak out against FGM may face social stigma and be branded as disobedient or rebellious. Many people are forced to follow the practice out of fear of these outcomes. In certain communities, a woman who has not undergone FGM is prohibited from speaking in public, going grocery shopping, or even fetching water. To avoid FGM, she has to flee from her community.

3. Control of Female Sexuality: FGM is occasionally employed to regulate female sexuality. Some groups think it lessens a woman's propensity for promiscuity and sexual desire. This stems from damaging gender stereotypes and norms. FGM is believed to preserve a girl's virginity and purity by reducing her sexual desire and ability to engage in premarital or extramarital sex. In societies where premarital sex is strictly prohibited, FGM is seen as a safeguard against promiscuity. FGM is a crime against female sexuality that aims to emotionally and sexually subjugate women.

4. Belief in Health and Hygiene: According to certain communities, FGM encourages women to practise better hygiene and health, which lowers their risk of infections and complications during childbirth. The idea that women must undergo FGM in order

to become pregnant is widely held. In fact, FGM does not improve fertility but can cause infertility and an increased risk of childbirth complications and even deaths in newborns. This misguided belief sustains the practice.

It's important to note that FGM is internationally recognised as a violation of human rights, as it can lead to severe physical and psychological consequences for those who undergo it.

How FGM is related to human rights:

1. Violation of the Right to Health: FGM can result in severe physical and psychological health consequences, including pain, infections, complications during childbirth, and long-term psychological trauma. It violates a woman's right to the highest attainable standard of physical and mental health, which is protected under various human rights treaties.
2. Violation of the Right to Be Free from Torture and Cruel, Inhuman, or Degrading Treatment: Female genital mutilation causes great pain and suffering to girls and women, and according to international human rights law, it is a kind of torture or cruel, inhuman, or degrading treatment. The United Nations and various other international organisations have repeatedly stated that FGM violates this right.
3. Violation of the Right to Life: In some cases, FGM can lead to fatal complications, especially during childbirth. While not all forms of FGM result in death, the practice still poses a risk to the right to life, as it increases the chances of life-threatening health issues.
4. Violation of the Right to Non-Discrimination:

The majority of victims of FGM are women and girls. It has its roots in discriminatory cultural practices and gender inequality. It is a part of the larger endeavour to advance gender equality and nondiscrimination to safeguard women and girls from FGM.
5. Violation of the Rights of the Child: FGM is often performed on girls, sometimes at a very young age, which is a clear violation of the rights of the child. It subjects them to physical and psychological harm without their informed consent.
6. Violation of the Right to Freedom from Violence and Harm: FGM is an act of violence against women and girls, and it undermines their physical and mental well-being. It violates the right to be free from violence and harm, which is a fundamental human right.
7. Violation of the Right to Informed Consent: Usually, the person having FGM is not given their free and informed permission to the procedure. Human rights are fundamentally based on informed consent, and FGM violates this right because it lacks consent.

The fight against FGM involves the implementation of global agreements and treaties, including the United Nations Convention on the Elimination of All Forms of Discrimination Against Women (CEDAW) and the Convention on the Rights of the Child. Numerous nations have adopted legislation to outlaw and penalise FGM. Non-governmental organisations and champions of human rights are actively engaged in efforts to raise awareness and encourage the abandonment of this harmful practice. The human rights framework serves as a crucial instrument in combating FGM, underscoring the significance of upholding the rights and dignity of all individuals, regardless of their gender.

According to Jenifer, a traditional birth attendant in Tangulbei, Kenya, "There are three sorrows of womanhood. The first is when a girl has her genitalia cut... the second is when she is married and has to have her vagina opened... the third is when she gives birth."

Female Genital Mutilation exerts profound and extensive impacts on the physical and psychological health of women and girls who experience it. While long-term complications may manifest during childbirth and result in sexual dysfunction, the immediate effects include pain and trauma. The psychological effects are just as harmful. Addressing the fallout from FGM requires a comprehensive approach that incorporates medical intervention, education, and cultural awareness to end this destructive practice and support survivors in their journey towards mental and physical healing.

PHYSICAL EFFECTS OF FGM

Short-term physical effects of FGM:

1. Pain and Immediate Discomfort: Most girls and women who undergo FGM experience severe pain, bleeding, and shock immediately after the procedure.
2. Risk of Infection: The risk of infection is increased by the fact that FGM is frequently carried out in unhygienic settings with non-sterile instruments. Complications such as septicemia or abscesses can result from infections.
3. Hemorrhage: Excessive bleeding during and after the procedure is common and can be life-threatening.
4. Urinary Problems: FGM can result in difficulty urinating due to pain and the obstruction of urine flow. This can lead to urinary tract infections.
5. Wound Healing Issues: Poor wound healing may result in the formation of scar tissue, which can be problematic in the long term.

Long-term physical effects of FGM:

1. Scar Tissue: The formation of scar tissue can cause

long-term discomfort and pain, particularly during sexual intercourse and childbirth.
2. Sexual Dysfunction: FGM can lead to sexual problems, including reduced sexual desire, pain during intercourse, and difficulties in achieving sexual satisfaction. This can significantly impact a woman's overall quality of life.
3. Obstetric Complications: FGM increases the risk of complications during childbirth, including obstructed labour, prolonged labour, and the need for emergency cesarean sections. These complications can pose significant risks to both the mother and the baby.
4. Infertility: In some cases, severe FGM can lead to infertility due to the obstruction of the reproductive tract.
5. Infection and Hygiene Issues: Women who have had FGM are concerned about recurring infections, especially in places with poor sanitation and little access to healthcare.

FGM raises the chance of women needing further operations in the future. For example, for a girl who has had her vaginal opening sealed or narrowed, she will need this to be cut open later to allow for sexual intercourse and childbirth. Sometimes a woman's vagina will be cut open and stitched closed again several times, meaning she goes through the pain again and again and is continually at risk (The problems with FGM explained, Action Aid).

Due to the sensitive nature of this topic, images are not included as they might be distressing. If you are interested, scan below to view real-life outcomes of FGM and get more information from the National Library of Medicine database.

PSYCHOLOGICAL EFFECTS OF FGM

Short-term psychological effects of FGM:

1. Physical and emotional trauma: The immediate pain, bleeding, and shock from the procedure can lead to severe emotional trauma. It can be a frightening and painful experience.
2. Anxiety and depression: Many girls and women who undergo FGM experience anxiety and depression as a result of the trauma they have endured.
3. Post-traumatic stress disorder (PTSD): Some individuals develop PTSD, which is characterised by flashbacks, nightmares, and severe anxiety triggered by reminders of the trauma.
4. Trust issues: Because FGM is frequently carried out by family members or neighbours, people may feel betrayed by those they believed to be protecting them, which can cause a breakdown in trust.
5. Difficulty in intimate relationships: FGM can cause physical and emotional problems during sexual intercourse, which can lead to difficulties in intimate relationships and marital issues.

Long-term psychological effects of FGM:

1. Chronic pain: Some women experience chronic pain and discomfort due to the scarring and damage caused by FGM, leading to ongoing physical and emotional distress.
2. Sexual dysfunction: FGM can result in sexual dysfunction, including pain during sexual activity, which can affect relationships and sexual satisfaction in the long run.
3. Gynaecological problems: FGM increases the risk of gynaecological issues, such as recurrent infections, infertility, and complications during childbirth, which can contribute to long-term psychological distress.
4. Low self-esteem and self-worth: The physical and emotional consequences of FGM can contribute to low self-esteem and feelings of inadequacy.
5. Stigmatisation and social isolation: Stigmatisation and social isolation among women who have experienced female genital mutilation can lead to long-term psychological distress.
6. Mental health issues: FGM can contribute to long-term mental health issues, such as anxiety, depression, and complex trauma.
7. In many communities, girls are forced to drop out of school after FGM and forced into early marriage.

According to the trauma psychologist and healer Peter Levine, who speaks about the tyranny of the past, "certain shocks to the organism can alter a person's biological, psychological and social equilibrium to such a degree that the memory of one particular event comes to taint, and dominate, all other experiences, spoiling an appreciation of the present moment" (Levin, Trauma and Memory, 2015).

A GEOGRAPHICAL APPROACH OF FGM

The origins of female genital mutilation are shrouded in uncertainty. Nevertheless, historical evidence indicates its practice among the Pharaohs in ancient Egypt. According to the UN, it was also prevalent in certain regions of Africa, the Philippines, among select tribes in the Upper Amazon, the Arunda tribe in Australia, some early Romans, and Arabs.

During the 19th century, gynaecologists in both Britain and the USA employed this procedure to address various ailments, such as epilepsy, hysteria, mental disorders, and depression, and to curb female masturbation, nymphomania, and even female homosexuality. It is important to note that such practices lacked any medical validity.

An estimated 200 million girls and women are currently living with FGM, with an additional 8,000 girls at risk every day, approximately 3 million girls per year (UNICEF, 2019). According to WHO, treatment of the health complications of FGM is estimated to cost health systems US$ 1.4 billion per year, a number expected to rise.

FGM is not limited to any one area of the world; it is practiced in many different parts of the world, including Africa, the Middle East, some parts of Asia, and Europe. There can be notable differences in the prevalence and type of FGM both within and between nations. It is crucial to note that FGM is not associated with any specific religion, as it is practised by individuals of both Muslim and Christian faiths in certain areas.

Here is a general overview of where FGM is prevalent:

1. Africa: FGM is most commonly practised in Africa, with prevalence rates varying from country to country. Nations like Somalia, Sudan, Guinea, and Djibouti have some of the highest prevalence rates. Somalia has one of the highest rates of FGM, where 98% of 15-19-year-old girls have been cut.
2. Middle East: FGM is also practised in some Middle Eastern countries, such as Egypt and Yemen. In these regions, the prevalence of FGM can differ depending on cultural and social factors.
3. Asia: Parts of Asia, including Indonesia, Malaysia, and some communities in India and Pakistan, have reported instances of FGM. It's essential to understand that FGM is not widespread across Asia and varies by region and community.
4. Europe: 16 European countries have reported FGM cases because of the migration of communities from countries where this practice is prevalent.

AFRICA

There is a Somali poem called "The Three Sorrows of Women" according to which "Love hurts three times: when you are cut, when you marry and when you give birth."

According to the tradition, if the little girl does not scream, cry, or show pain, she is also worthy in addition to being brave. Worthy to be a woman, wife, mother.

FGM is prevalent in 30 countries in Africa.

I will list the countries in Africa and the percentages of the female population that undergo FGM (the figures are as listed by the organization Equality Now).

Egypt 87%, Sudan 87%, Eritrea 83%, Ethiopia 65%, Djibouti 94%, Somalia 98%, Sierra Leone 86%, Mali 89%, Guinea 95%, Burkina Faso 76%, Gambia 76%, Mauritania 67%, Guinea-Bissau 45%, Liberia 44%, Chad 38%, Cote d'Ivoire 37%, Senegal 24%, C.R.A 24%, Kenya 21%, Nigeria 19%, Tanzania 10%, Benin 9%, Gana 4%, Togo 3%, Niger 2%, Zambia 1% and Uganda 1%.

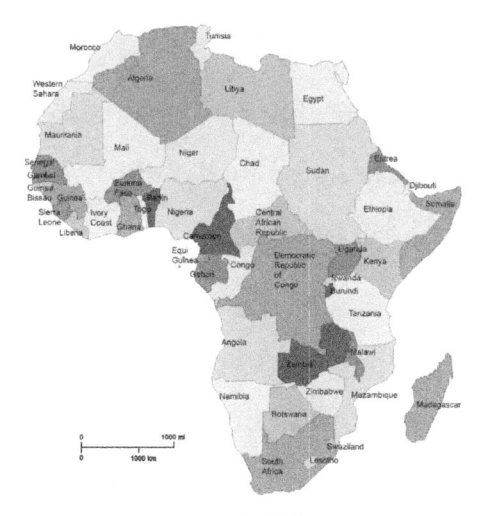

Map of Africa

FGM is taking place in the Democratic Republic of the Congo, Libya, Malawi, South Sudan, South Africa and Zimbabwe, but no prevalence estimates are available.

The 50% of FGM women live in Egypt, Ethiopia and Indonesia.

In numerous West African societies, the clitoris has been viewed as a source and bearer of malevolent forces for centuries. The general consensus is that women's clitoris is a remnant of male anatomy that should be removed because it is seen as impure and dangerous for men. Men have a fear that the clitoris, like the penis, will grow larger, so they try not to touch it in order to avoid becoming sexually impotent. Meanwhile, women harbour the belief that if a newborn's head comes into contact with the clitoris during childbirth, the child will perish. Some men even entertain the notion that engaging in intimacy with an unclean woman will result in their penis being ensnared by her clitoris.

A fascinating legend from the Dogon tribe in West Africa's Mali gives this viewpoint a cultural context. Dogon mythology states that a child is born with both male and female characteristics. In this context, the clitoris is considered the male element in a girl. At the same time, the foreskin is viewed as the female element in a boy. The myth recounts that the supreme god Ama, without a husband, transformed the earth into his spouse. But Ama was unable to mate with her in order to have children because of the difficulty posed by termite nests all over the ground. As a result, he had to chop down the termite nests.

Some information about FGM in Egypt:

According to the Egyptian Family Health Survey (EFHS) 2021, 86 percent of Egyptian married women between the ages of 15 and 49 have undergone FGM. In Egypt, FGM is performed by men.

The practice of FGM, or FGM, is widespread in Egypt, where it is highly prevalent and has a centuries-long historical legacy. Although women's views on circumcision have positively changed, FGM still poses a serious threat in spite of concerted efforts to address it.

Recent data from the EFHS in 2021 indicates a noteworthy decline, with only 13% of mothers expressing an intention to circumcise their daughters in the future, in contrast to the approximately 35% reported in the Demographic and Health Survey (DHS) of 2014.

In Egypt, FGM encompasses various degrees of cutting, ranging from the removal of the clitoral hood to the more severe form involving the excision of the clitoris and labia, coupled with the suturing of the vaginal opening (infibulation).

The practice of FGM in Egypt is driven by a complex interplay of cultural, social, and religious factors. Some communities view it as a rite of passage or a means to regulate female sexuality. In contrast, others associate it with religious or hygiene considerations despite the absence of any religious foundation for the practice in Islam. Despite positive shifts in attitudes, the persistence of FGM underscores the ongoing need for comprehensive efforts to eradicate this harmful practice.

Legislation has been enacted in Egypt to combat FGM. In June 2008, the government incorporated FGM/C as a criminal offence in the Penal Code, rendering it illegal. The law mandates a minimum custodial sentence of three months and a maximum of two years or an alternative penalty ranging from 1,000 to 5,000 Egyptian pounds (LE). In 2021, the Egyptian parliament passed amendments raising the minimum and maximum terms of imprisonment for FGM offences. The changes stipulated that medical personnel who perform genital mutilation, such as physicians and nurses, could be imprisoned for a maximum of 10 to 15 years. Notwithstanding these legal actions, anti-FGM laws are not consistently enforced, which permits the practice to continue in some areas.

Some information about FGM in Somalia:

FGM is widespread in Somalia, with estimates indicating that nearly 98% of females aged 5-11 have experienced Type III (infibulations), the most brutal form of genital cutting. This practice is deeply ingrained in Somali culture and is commonly regarded as a rite of passage.

The predominant form of FGM/C in Somalia is Type III, also known as infibulation or "Pharaonic circumcision" in the local context. This severe form involves the removal of all external genitalia, with the vaginal opening sewn shut.

Cultural and social beliefs often drive the performance of FGM, seen as a means to safeguard a girl's chastity, modesty, and purity. In certain communities, FGM is deemed a prerequisite for marriage, believed to enhance a girl's social acceptance and respect. Typically, FGM procedures are conducted by designated individuals in the community, often elderly individuals, predominantly women, or traditional birth attendants.

The most famous Somalian activist is **Waris Dirie**.

Waris Dirie, born in 1965 in Galcaio, Somalia, is renowned as a Somali fashion model, author, and advocate for women's rights. She is particularly recognised for her dedicated work towards eradicating FGM, also referred to as female circumcision. Raised in a large nomadic family near Somalia's border with Ethiopia, Dirie is one of 12 siblings.

FGM is not expressly illegal or punishable in Somalia, despite the Provisional 2012 Constitution of the country clearly denouncing the "cruel and degrading customary practice" of circumcising girls, comparing it to torture, and outlawing such practices.

Some information about FGM in Ethiopia.

In Ethiopia, the practice of female genital mutilation/

cutting (FGM/C) is deeply rooted in tradition, culture, and beliefs, as well as in community values pertaining to gender, femininity, and sexuality of women. The prevalence of this practice varies significantly across communities due to regional differences and the complex interplay between FGM/C and cultural and religious beliefs, as highlighted by Mehari *et al.* (2020). Individual and community knowledge and attitudes towards the practice, educational attainment, geographic locations within the nation, and, to some extent, religious influences are factors influencing the prevalence (Abebe *et al.*, 2020).

In the Somali region of Ethiopia, the practice of FGM/C is often motivated by the desire to enhance marriageability, as noted by Abathun *et al.* (2016). A girl who has not undergone the procedure may be perceived as ineligible for marriage, creating strong social pressures for adherence to this cultural norm. Persistent fears of community stigma and the potential social consequences, including severe social sanctions on their households, drive mothers to conform to the practice (Mehari *et al.*, 2020). Failure to comply is seen as bringing shame to the family and jeopardising the standing of any potential future husband for their daughters (Elamin and Mason-Jones, 2020; Mehari *et al.*, 2020). Uncut girls may encounter difficulties in finding a husband within the Somali cultural setting (Mehari *et al.*, 2020).

Moreover, the fear of being ostracised by peers compels girls to take matters into their own hands, organising their own circumcision to assume responsibility for protecting their families from potential legal and social sanctions, as highlighted by Boyden *et al.* (2013).

Somalia, Guinea and Djibouti remain the countries with the highest rate of FGM/C in the world. While at the same time, the percentage of girls undergoing FGM/C decreased in thirty other countries, including Liberia, Burkina Faso and Kenya.

The latest approach in African nations involves affluent families sending girls to Europe for FGM/C procedures performed by qualified doctors to minimise the risk of fatalities. However, this does not justify the practice in any manner.

A worldwide plan to end this cruel practice was unveiled in 2010 by the UN and the World Health Organisation. The UN General Assembly then adopted a resolution in 2012 with the goal of outlawing FGM.

As of 2013, FGM is prohibited in 26 African countries, yet enforcement of the law seems lax, underscoring the significance of information as the sole tool in addressing this issue.

The Maputo Protocol, formally titled "The Protocol to the African Charter on Human and Peoples' Rights on the Rights of Women in Africa," was endorsed by the African Union in 2003 as a supplementary protocol to the African Charter on Human and Peoples' Rights. To date, 53 African countries have endorsed the Convention, with 28 having formally ratified it.

The Protocol's Article 5 lists FGM as a harmful practice. In order to inform the public about the dangers of FGM and other harmful practices, this particular article supports the creation of awareness campaigns and the implementation of focused support services.

ASIA-PACIFIC REGION

Some information about FGM in Indonesia.

FGM, traditionally thought to be primarily practiced in sub-Saharan Africa and the Middle East, has been revealed to be prevalent in Indonesia, according to a recent report by the United Nations Children's Fund.

In Indonesia, girls commonly undergo FGC Type I or Type IV, with instances of what is termed as "symbolic" cutting. Various practices are reported, including the application of iodine or turmeric on the clitoris, nicking, pricking, and even the use of a chicken to peck at a girl's genitals.

Local practices in Indonesia involve actions that cause harm to female genitalia, such as cutting or slicing a small part of the clitoral hood, pinching with metal, piercing with a hypodermic needle, and rubbing with a blunt object like metal, plant, or pottery shard (kreweng). Unconventional methods include spreading rice grains over the vaginal surface to be pecked at by a rooster. These actions are considered as ways to cause injury to female genitals, accompanied by bleeding, signifying the fulfilment of the obligation to be circumcised. In Indonesian, this practice is commonly referred to as "sunat perempuan" (female circumcision), literally meaning an action of cutting or injuring certain parts of female genitals (One Decade of Indonesia's Efforts in Eradication of the practice of FGM/C, UNFPA in partnership with Canada, Lies Marcoes, UNFPA 2023).

Surprisingly, Indonesia does not have a national law prohibiting FGM/FGC. Small, symbolic clitoris incisions are allowed by customary law. After Mauritania and Mali, Indonesia has the third-highest prevalence rate in the world, at 49 percent. According to a 2013 study by Indonesian Basic Health Research, 51% of girls in the country up to the age of 11 had undergone circumcision.

Some statistics:

AUSTRALIA Indirect estimates indicate that there are 53,088 survivors of FGM/C living in Australia.

BRUNEI DARUSSALAM The Government of Brunei has affirmed the practice of Type I FGM/C within the country. While specific prevalence rates are not available, FGM/C is acknowledged as widespread within the Malay community, constituting a significant portion of Brunei's population.

INDIA FGM/C is practised within the Bohra community and a Sunni Muslim sect in Kerala, India. The Bohra population is estimated at around 1 million, with a 2018 study indicating a 75% prevalence of FGM/C among daughters of respondents in the sample. The Bohra community practices Type I FGM/C, locally known as "khatna" or "khafz," involving the cutting of the clitoral hood and/or clitoris.

MALAYSIA The Malaysian government estimates that 83-85% of Muslim baby girls undergo circumcision by medical professionals in private clinics. Research studies also suggest a high prevalence of FGM/C, particularly Type I/Type IV, involving the cutting/pricking of the clitoral hood and/or clitoris, often performed on babies aged 1-2 months.

MALDIVES National prevalence data indicates a 13% prevalence of FGM/C among women and girls aged 15-49 in the Maldives but only 1% among girls aged 0-14. Anecdotal evidence suggests that Type IV FGM/C, characterised by small cuts to the genitals, is the primary practice in the Maldives.

NEW ZEALAND: While anecdotal evidence points to survivors of FGM/C from diaspora communities in New Zealand, there is no reliable estimate available.

PAKISTAN: FGM/C occurs within the Bohra community in Pakistan, comprising around 100,000 people. Despite the absence of prevalence estimates, Type I FGM/C is practised, involving the cutting of the clitoral hood and/or clitoris, referred to as "khatna" or "khafz" within the Bohra community.

PHILIPPINES: 54 FGM/C is only practiced in a few isolated areas of the Philippines, mostly among Muslim populations in the Mindanao region. The majority of this practice, called pag-sunnat or turi, is classified as Type IV, though there are sporadic instances of Type I, especially among the Meranaos.

SINGAPORE: FGM/C is acknowledged in the Malay Muslim community in Singapore, constituting approximately 15% of the total population. However, no prevalence estimates are available. Malays typically practice Type I/Type IV FGM/C, involving cutting/pricking of the clitoral hood and/or clitoris, in a procedure known as "sunat perempuan."

SRI LANKA: FGM/C is known to occur among the Moor, Malay, and Bohra communities in Sri Lanka, with no prevalence estimates available. The practised type is usually Type I/Type IV FGM/C, involving cutting/pricking of the clitoral hood and/or clitoris.

THAILAND: FGM/C is practised by Muslim communities in

Thailand, constituting 5-8% of the total population, mainly concentrated in the southern provinces of Yala, Narathiwat, and Pattani. Type I/Type IV FGM/C, involving cutting/pricking of the clitoral hood and/or clitoris, is known to be practised in a procedure called 'sunat' or 'sunat perempuan.'

MIDDLE EAST

The Arab region hosts 50 million cases of FGM, constituting a quarter of the global instances. Notably, the Holy Quran remains silent on FGM, lacking any explicit reference. There is no consensus (Ijma') on a specific legal ruling and no accepted analogy (Qiyas) regarding the practice.

In the Middle East, Saudi Arabia's northern region, Iraq, and southern Jordan are the main locations for FGM. Reports of similar incidents have also come from the United Arab Emirates, Syria, and Qatar. FGM is most common in small ethnic communities where it is maintained as a custom. There can be differences in the frequency and intensity of FGM practices in rural and urban settings.

Yemen records that 19% of women and girls aged 15-49 have experienced FGM. Sudan initially legislated against Type III FGM in 1946, but it was widely ignored. In 1983, it was entirely removed with the advent of Sharia law. Despite subsequent efforts, such as the National Child Act of 2009, FGM was not criminalised in Sudan until 2020.

Historically, Saudi Arabia, due to government restrictions and a small immigrant population, was not thought to witness widespread FGM/C. However, a recent survey revealed that 18.2% of women in a Saudi obstetrics and gynaecology clinic self-reported having undergone FGM/C during childhood.

In Bangladesh, it is crucial to emphasise that FGM still occurs in the country, primarily linked to the beliefs and customs of Muslim communities. These communities argue in favour of continuing the practice, citing perceived "medical benefits" associated with female circumcision.

In Pakistan, there are no legal or administrative measures in place to prevent FGM practices. The absence of specific laws addressing FGM is due to the underreporting and lack of recognition of its occurrence, possibly because the issue is discreetly practised within a small religious community.

Oman ranks among the countries with the highest prevalence of FGM globally, surpassing 80 per cent, according to the UN. However, women from the capital, Muscat, appear to be less affected.

In Bahrain, although there have been reported cases in the past, FGM/C is not currently practised. Prosecution under

Article 337 of the Penal Code is possible for FGM/C, treating it as assault. Notably, marital rape is not criminalised in the Penal Code.

Kuwait lacks a law criminalising or prohibiting FGM/C, despite the prevalence of the practice.

In Iraq, a religious decree has been issued mandating FGM for all girls and women aged 11 to 46 in and around Mosul. This decree impacts approximately 4 million girls and women in the region.

EUROPE

The European Union projects that approximately 600,000 women and girls are grappling with the repercussions of female genital mutilation within its borders. In addition, 180,000 more women and girls in 13 European countries run the immediate risk of being subjected to this harmful practice. Beyond diaspora communities, data suggests that FGM occurs in Russia and Georgia in non-diaspora communities. Notably, FGM has been specifically targeted by laws or legal provisions in 16 European countries; Georgia recently joined them by enacting a law against this harmful practice.

Some statistics:

AUSTRIA – Indirect estimates indicate 7,036 women and girls who have undergone FGM/C.

BELGIUM – Indirect estimates indicate 17,575 women and girls who have undergone FGM/C, with a further 8,342 at risk.

BULGARIA – Indirect estimates indicate 31 women and girls who have undergone FGM/C.

CROATIA – Indirect estimates indicate 112 women and girls who have undergone FGM/C.

CYPRUS – Indirect estimates indicate 1,301 women and girls who have undergone FGM/C, with a further 132 at risk.

CZECH REPUBLIC – Indirect estimates indicate 312 women and girls who have undergone FGM/C.

DENMARK – Indirect estimates indicate 7,910 women and girls who have undergone FGM/C.

ESTONIA – Indirect estimates indicate 8 women and girls who have undergone FGM/C.

FINLAND – Indirect estimates indicate 10,254 women and girls who have undergone FGM/C, with a further 3,075 at risk.

FRANCE – Indirect estimates indicate 125,000 women and girls who have undergone FGM/C, with a further 44,106 at risk. In France, in article 312 par.3 of the Criminal Code, there is a need for proportional use of the terms mutilation and excision. The above article was applied proportionally in 1983 in the Cour de Cassation for the first time. At the time, clitoridectomy was labelled a "cultural crime" (delit culturel).

GEORGIA – Type I FGM/C is practised by the Avar community

(a small community in Georgia with a population of around 3000).

GERMANY- In Germany, indirect estimates are suggesting that 70,218 women and girls have experienced FGM/C, and an additional 17,691 are considered at risk. The country's legal framework, specifically articles 223 et seq. of the Criminal Code, grants judges the authority to impose prison sentences ranging from 1 to 10 years for individuals found guilty of committing FGM. The severity of the punishment may be influenced by categorising the act as either grievous bodily harm or attempted murder in certain cases.

GREECE – Indirect estimates indicate 15,249 women and girls who have undergone FGM/C, with a further 748 at risk.

HUNGARY – Indirect estimates indicate 396 women and girls who have undergone FGM/C.

IRELAND – Indirect estimates indicate 5,790 women and girls who have undergone FGM/C, with a further 1,632 at risk.

ITALY – Indirect estimates indicate 70,469 women and girls who have undergone FGM/C, with a further 18,339 at risk.

LATVIA – Indirect estimates indicate 5 women and girls who have undergone FGM/C.

LUXEMBOURG – Indirect estimates indicate 379 women and

girls who have undergone FGM/C.

MALTA – Indirect estimates indicate 565 women and girls who have undergone FGM/C, with a further 279 at risk.

NETHERLANDS – Indirect estimates indicate 41,000 women and girls who have undergone FGM/C, with a further 4,200 at risk.

NORWAY – Indirect estimates indicate 17,058 women and girls who have undergone FGM/C.

POLAND – Indirect estimates indicate 207 women and girls who have undergone FGM/C.

PORTUGAL – Indirect estimates indicate 6,576 women and girls who have undergone FGM/C, with a further 1,365 at risk.

ROMANIA – Indirect estimates indicate 79 women and girls who have undergone FGM/C.

RUSSIA – In Russia, the Avar community in East Dagestan practices FGM/C. Type I FGM/C is predominant, with the Andi people exhibiting instances of both clitoral and labial removal (Type II FGM/C). Approximately 1,240 girls are estimated to be at risk of experiencing FGM/C annually.

SLOVAKIA – Indirect estimates indicate 57 women and girls who have undergone FGM/C.

SLOVENIA – Indirect estimates indicate 69 women and girls

who have undergone FGM/C.

SPAIN – Indirect estimates indicate 15,907 women and girls who have undergone FGM/C.

SWEDEN – Indirect assessments suggest that 38,939 women and girls in Sweden have experienced FGM/C, with an additional 11,145 at risk. Since 1982, Sweden has enacted a law prohibiting "any form of intervention on the external genitalia resulting in cutting off or permanently altering them."

SWITZERLAND-In Switzerland, indirect estimates indicate that 14,700 women and girls have undergone FGM/C. Article 122 of the Penal Code in Switzerland declares that "anyone who mutilates one of the members or organs crucial for the proper functioning of another person's body shall be subject to a penalty of ten or more years of compulsory community service or imprisonment ranging from six months to five years."

Within the European Union, several essential instruments have been established to combat the harrowing practice of FGM in Europe. These include:

    a. The European Commission Communication on the eradication of FGM, endorsed by both the European

Parliament and the Council of the European Union.

b. The Istanbul Convention.

UNITED KINGDOM

Approximately 137,000 women and girls have experienced FGM/C, and an additional 67,300 are at risk, according to indirect estimates. London holds the highest national prevalence among cities, affecting an estimated 2.1% of women. In the UK, the age group most commonly subjected to FGM is between 5 and 9 years old.

The summer school vacation, which is referred to as the "cutting season" informally, is a time when a significant number of FGM cases occur. This schedule enables the girls to heal before going back to school.

Signs that FGM might be imminent or has occurred include:

- A female relative, such as a mother, sister, or aunt, has undergone FGM.
- A relative or an individual known for practising FGM visiting from abroad.
- A family planning an extended overseas holiday or visit to family abroad.

- Observable behaviours in a girl, such as talking about a special 'ceremony,' unexpected or prolonged absence from school, withdrawal, academic struggles, spending an extended time in the bathroom, and appearing uncomfortable while sitting, walking, or standing.

Legal Framework in the UK:

FGM became prohibited in the UK in 1985 through the enactment of the Prohibition of Female Circumcision Act. Subsequent legislative measures, such as the Female Genital Mutilation Act 2003 and the Serious Crime Act 2015, further strengthened and extended this prohibition.

The legislation criminalises the performance of FGM and any involvement in aiding, abetting, or assisting in its commission, whether within the UK or abroad.

Individuals convicted of FGM offences face penalties that may include a maximum prison sentence of up to 14 years.

In particular, The Legal Framework

FGM offences are set out in the FGM Act 2003 as amended by the Serious Crime Act 2015.

Definitions under the FGM Act 2003

- The term "girl" includes "woman": section 6(1).
- A United Kingdom national is an individual who is:
  - ➢ a British citizen, a British overseas territories citizen, a British national (overseas) or a British overseas citizen;
  - ➢ a person who, under the British Nationality Act 1981, is a British subject; or
  - ➢ a British protected person within the meaning of that Act: section 6(2).

A United Kingdom resident is "an individual who is habitually resident in the UK". The term "habitually resident" covers a person's ordinary residence instead of a short temporary stay in a country. To be habitually resident in the UK, it may not be necessary for all, or any, of the period of residence here to be lawful. Whether a person is habitually resident in the UK should be determined by the facts of the case.

Offences

There are four FGM offences under the FGM Act 2003:

- the primary offence of FGM: section 1
- assisting a girl to mutilate her own genitals: section 2
- assisting a non-UK person to mutilate a girl's genitals overseas: section 3; and
- failing to protect a girl from the risk of FGM: section 3A.

Offence of FGM – section 1

It is a criminal offence to "excise, infibulate or otherwise mutilate" the whole or any part of a girl's labia majora, labia minora or clitoris: section 1(1) FGM Act 2003.

This is an offence even where the act is done outside the United Kingdom, where it is done by a United Kingdom national or resident, by virtue of section 4 of the FGM Act 2003.

There is no statutory definition or judicial consideration of the conduct elements of the offence. Each is to be given its ordinary and natural meaning:

- "excise" means to cut out/off, cut away, extract, remove;
- "infibulate" means to close off or obstruct (including suture of) the genitalia, and it is submitted, therefore,

includes re-infibulation; and

- "mutilate" (according to the Oxford English Dictionary) means "to deprive... of the use of a limb or bodily organ, by dismemberment or otherwise; to cut off or destroy (a limb or organ); to wound severely; or to inflict violent or disfiguring injury on". "Disfigure" means "to spoil the appearance of", and "disfiguring injury" must be interpreted accordingly. The definition does not suggest that the disfiguring injury should be permanent; any procedure which temporarily spoils the appearance of the genitalia is, therefore, capable of falling within the definition of "disfiguring injury" and potentially of "mutilation".

Whether the particular procedure amounts to excision, infibulation or mutilation of the genitalia is a question of fact which should be established by medical and/or other expert evidence.

It follows from the above that the forms of FGM which fall within the WHO Type IV classification may or may not amount to "mutilation" for the purposes of the commission of an offence under section 1(1) of the FGM Act 2003. Much will depend on the case's particular circumstances and whether the evidence taken as a whole demonstrates mutilation. Prosecutors must ensure that the evidence is focused on one or more of the three forms of FGM provided for by the FGM Act 2003.

The following medical procedures are exempted from the offence (sections 1(2)-1(5) FGM Act 2003):

- A surgical operation on a girl is necessary for her physical and mental health if performed by a registered medical practitioner.
- In determining whether an operation is necessary for the mental health of a girl, it is immaterial whether she or any other person believes that the operation is required as a matter of custom or ritual.
- A surgical operation on a girl who is in any stage of labour or has just given birth for purposes connected with the labour or birth if performed by a registered medical practitioner or a registered midwife for a person undergoing a course of training to become such practitioner or midwife.

If the same medical procedures are carried out outside of the United Kingdom by an individual performing the duties of a registered midwife or registered medical practitioner, as the case may be, they are also exempt.

Assisting a girl to mutilate her own genitals – section 2

Self-mutilation is not an offence, but it is an offence to assist a girl to do so. A person is guilty of an offence if it is proved that:

- a girl has excised, infibulated or otherwise mutilated the whole or any part of her own labia majora, labia minora or clitoris, and
- the suspect has aided, abetted, counselled or procured this.

This is an offence even where any act is done outside the United Kingdom, where it is done by a United Kingdom national or resident, by virtue of section 4 of the FGM Act 2003. Thus, the act of FGM by the girl may take place anywhere in the world and/or the act of aiding, abetting, counselling or procuring it may take place anywhere in the world, provided that the act is done by a United Kingdom national or resident. Aiding, abetting, counselling or procuring can occur by many means, including online.

Assisting a non-UK person to mutilate a girl's genitals overseas - section 3

A person is guilty of an offence if it is proved that:

- excision, infibulation or otherwise mutilation of the whole or any part of a girl's labia major, labia minora or clitoris has taken place, and
- the girl is a United Kingdom national or a United Kingdom resident, and
- this was done by a person who is not a United Kingdom national or a United Kingdom resident and
- this act of FGM took place outside the United Kingdom, and
- the suspect aided, abetted, counselled or procured this.

Sections 1 and 2 of the FGM Act 2003 address a suspect doing FGM themselves, or a girl committing the act and the suspect aiding, abetting, procuring or counselling this: in cases where the act and/or the aiding/abetting/counselling/procuring is by a United Kingdom national or resident, it is an offence irrespective of where either of those acts was done in the world. Section 3 on the other hand, covers an individual who performs FGM who is not a resident or national of the

United Kingdom and who does so anywhere in the world; however, in cases where the victim is a resident or national of the United Kingdom, anyone who aids and abets in the FGM act will be held accountable.

Failing to protect a girl from risk of genital mutilation – section 3A

If an offence under sections 1, 2 or 3 of the FGM Act 2003 is committed against a girl under the age of 16, then each person who is responsible for her will be potentially liable if they knew, or ought to have known, that there was a significant risk of FGM being carried out but did not take reasonable steps to prevent it from happening. Note that "under 16" is the threshold for this offence, as distinct from "under 18" which has been used for the duty to report and the public interest factors elsewhere in this guidance.

This offence can be committed wholly or partly outside the United Kingdom by a person who is a United Kingdom national or resident: neither the culpable failure nor the FGM need to take place within the jurisdiction.

Responsibility under section 3A of the FGM Act 2003 arises in either of two situations:

- the person has parental responsibility for the girl and has frequent contact with her at the relevant time (when the FGM occurs). Frequent contact is treated as continuing if the girl temporarily stays elsewhere; or
- the person is aged 18 or over and has assumed, and not relinquished, responsibility for caring for the girl in the manner of a parent at the relevant time (when the FGM occurs).

It is a defence for a defendant to show that either:

- at the relevant time (when the FGM occurs), the defendant did not think that there was a significant risk of FGM being committed against the girl, and could not reasonably have been expected to be aware that there was any such risk; or
- the defendant took such steps as they could reasonably have been expected to take to protect the girl from being the victim of an FGM offence at the relevant time (when the FGM occurs).

There is an evidential burden on the defendant to raise these defences but, once raised, the prosecution must prove the contrary to the criminal standard of proof.

The facts of each case will determine what reasonable steps the defendant took to prevent the girl from becoming the victim of a FGM offence, should they choose to raise this defence. For example, the steps considered reasonable for a woman to take in the case where her overbearing and violent husband or another family member had arranged for FGM to be carried out on her daughter may well differ from those taken by a woman who is not subjected to those pressures. It is important to make an assessment on a case-by-case basis.

There may be clear evidence that a girl has been the subject of FGM, but more than one person in the household could be responsible. Prosecutors will consider the evidence that one person was responsible or whether a joint enterprise existed. Guidance on joint enterprise in these circumstances can be gained from the following cases:

R v Abbott (1955) 39 Cr.App.R. 141:

"If two people are jointly indicted for the commission of a crime and the evidence does not point to one rather than the other, and there is no evidence they were acting in concert, the jury ought to return a verdict of not guilty in the case of both as the prosecution have not proved the case."

R v Strudwick and Merry (1994) 99 Cr.App.R. 326:

lies told by one or other of the parents as to the cause of injury may support a prosecution case, but they do not, without more, make a positive case of the crime in question.

Where joint enterprise cannot be established, the prosecution should consider the evidence in support of the section 3A offence.

Those who have parental responsibility and how they can acquire it are set out in section 2 Children Act 1989. It includes, for example:

- a child's biological mother;
- a father who is married to the mother of the child when the child is born;
- an unmarried father registered on the child's birth certificate at the time of their birth;
- guardians; and
- persons named in a Child Arrangements Order.

The requirement for frequent contact is intended to ensure that a person who, in law, has parental responsibility for a girl but, in practice, has little or no contact with her would not be liable. For example, where the parents of a girl are separated and live apart, with one parent having little or no contact with their daughter, the parent with little or no contact would not be liable for the offence. Similarly, where an adult cares for a girl in the "manner of a parent", this is intended to ensure that a person looking after a girl for a very short period – such as a babysitter – would not be liable. Nor would it cover teachers working in their professional capacity. A person who assumes responsibility for caring for the girl in the manner of a parent can include, for example, grandparents with whom the girl has gone to stay for an extended summer holiday. In such circumstances, those persons with parental responsibility for the girl would continue to be liable for the offence as a result of section 3A (7) FGM Act 2003.

Extraterritoriality

When a suspect's culpable acts or FGM took place outside of England and Wales, the first thing to do is find out if they are a resident of the United Kingdom and carefully evaluate the evidence supporting this claim.

If the suspect is a UK national or resident, then the effect of section 4(1) FGM Act 2003 is that there is jurisdiction to prosecute, wherever in the world the following conduct is alleged to have taken place:

- the suspect personally committed the act of FGM on the victim

- the suspect aided or abetted the victim to commit FGM on herself
- the suspect aided or abetted another to commit FGM
- the suspect failed to protect a girl from FGM

In each case, the nationality or residence of the suspect provides for jurisdiction, wherever the culpable act (personally committing the offence; aiding or abetting a victim; aiding or abetting another; failing to protect) or the act of FGM occurred.

This is the case regardless of the nationality or residence of the victim.

In cases which involve a non-UK national or resident, in addition to liability for FGM undertaken in England and Wales, the following should be considered:

- if there is a substantial connection with the jurisdiction, if a substantial number of the activities constituting the crime take place within England and Wales, then the courts in England and Wales will have jurisdiction unless it can be argued, on a reasonable view, that the conduct ought to be dealt with by the courts of another country: *R v. Smith (Wallace Duncan) (No. 4)* [2004] 2 Cr.App.R.

17, CA.

- if a person:
  - agrees with another, or does an act or omission in pursuance of such an agreement, whilst in England or Wales,
  - that agreement is that a course of conduct would involve an act or an event outside England or Wales;
  - that act or event would amount to an FGM offence, contrary to the law of that country (thus requiring proof of the same);
  - that agreement would be triable as a section 1 conspiracy Criminal Law Act 1977 conspiracy, but for the extraterritorial element,

they commit an offence contrary to section 1A Criminal Law Act 1977. This offence requires the Attorney General's consent to prosecute. Prosecutors should consult Foreign and Commonwealth Office resources and/or the International Justice and Organised Crime Division to obtain the position and, if necessary, evidence of the actual legal position in the country concerned.

- a conspiracy contrary to section 1 Criminal Law Act 1977 to commit FGM in England and Wales can be tried in England and Wales even if the agreement is formed outside: Somchai Liangsiriprasert v Government of the United States of America [1991] 1 A.C. 225, PC; Sansom [1991] 2 Q.B. 130.

- if a person does act wholly or partly in England and Wales and knows or believes that what they anticipate might take place wholly or partly in a place outside England and Wales, and the anticipated offence is one contrary to the FGM Act 2003, that person is liable to prosecution for encouraging or assisting an offence pursuant to Part 2 and Schedule 4 of the Serious Crime Act 2007. This requires the Attorney General's consent to prosecute.

Other offences

If the trial issue, or one of the trial issues, identified is that the conduct did not amount to "mutilation", prosecutors should consider whether a charge contrary to section 18 or section 47 of the Offences Against the Person Act 1861 is more appropriate. Prosecutors should refer to offences against the person – charging standard legal guidance. These offences would apply where the evidence supports an allegation that:

- really serious bodily harm, or actual harm, was caused.

This need not be permanent or dangerous or have

lasting consequences. In assessing whether the harm was "grievous", account should be taken of the effect on the individual. This includes psychiatric but not psychological injury. The assessment of harm is for a jury, applying contemporary social standards: *Golding* [2014] EWCA Crim 889. *Bollom* [2003] EWCA Crim 2846 confirms that this is to be assessed with reference to the characteristics (including age and health) of the particular victim. "Actual harm" means injury which is more than transient and trifling or wounding, namely, a break in the continuity of the whole skin has occurred.

Equally, for an allegation contrary to section 3A FGM Act 2003 where the issue, or one of the issues identified, is "mutilation", then consideration may be given to the additional or alternative charge contrary at section 5, Domestic Violence, Crime and Victims Act 2004 of causing or allowing a child to suffer serious physical harm.

Anonymity of Victims

One of the reasons why victims of FGM may be reluctant to come forward and report the crime is because of the risk of being identified as a victim of such a personal and sensitive crime. Giving victims the protection that lifelong anonymity affords is intended to encourage more victims to come forward to report this crime.

Anonymity commences as soon as an allegation of FGM is made by the victim. This ensures that the victim is protected, whatever the outcome of the investigation or prosecution.

Section 4A and Schedule 1 of the FGM Act 2003 set out provisions for the anonymity of victims of FGM. The effect is to prohibit the publication of any matter that would likely lead members of the public to identify a person as the alleged victim of any offence under the FGM Act 2003. The prohibition lasts for the lifetime of the alleged victim. The prohibition covers not just immediate identifying information such as the name and address or a photograph of the alleged victim but any other information which, whether on its own or pieced together with other information, would likely lead members of the public to identify the alleged victim. If it is suggested that the defendants' identities be disclosed, it may be appropriate to restrict reporting of that information. Other information, like the scene of the incident or those who have taken on the victim's care afterward, may also be subject to reporting restrictions. "Publication" is broadly defined and would include traditional print media, broadcasting and social media such as Twitter or Facebook.

Exceptions to anonymity

There are two limited circumstances where the court may dis-apply the restrictions on publication:

- the first is where a person being tried for an FGM offence could have their defence substantially prejudiced if the restriction to prevent identification of the person against whom the allegation of FGM was committed is not lifted;
- the second is where preventing identification of the person against whom the allegation of FGM was committed could impose a substantial and unreasonable restriction on the reporting of the proceedings, and it is therefore considered in the public interest to remove this restriction.

Sentencing

A person guilty of an offence under sections 1, 2 and 3 of the FGM Act 2003 is liable:

- on conviction on indictment, to imprisonment for a term not exceeding 14 years or a fine (or both);
- on summary conviction, to imprisonment for a

term not exceeding six months or a fine (or both).
- A person guilty of an offence under section 3A of the FGM Act 2003 is liable in England and Wales:
- on conviction on indictment, to imprisonment for a term not exceeding 7 years or a fine (or both);
- on summary conviction, to imprisonment for a term not exceeding six months or a fine (or both).

A person guilty of an offence under section 4A of the FGM Act 2003 in England and Wales is liable to a fine on summary conviction.

a) First Successful Prosecution for Female Genital Mutilation.

A woman in London has been found guilty by a jury of committing female genital mutilation on her three-year-old daughter, marking the first conviction for this crime in the U.K. since its prohibition in 1985. The procedure was performed in their north London home in 2017 by a 37-year-old Ugandan woman. When the case went to trial, the Crown Prosecution Service proved that the girl had either had her genitalia removed completely or partially. About 12 hours after the sharp-tool incident, when the parents brought their severely injured child to the hospital, the situation was reported to the authorities.

In a statement, Inspector Allen Davis, the lead officer for FGM at the Metropolitan Police, emphasised the significance of this landmark conviction, expressing hope that it would send a clear message about the thorough investigation and prosecution of FGM cases. The parents, who cannot be identified for legal reasons, initially claimed the injuries resulted from a kitchen accident, stating the girl had fallen from a counter onto an open, metal-lined cupboard door. However, medical professionals determined that the injuries were inconsistent with such an accident and were indicative of FGM.

The parents, comprising the mother and a 43-year-old man from Ghana who is the girl's father, were initially arrested but later released on bail. Ultimately, the father was acquitted of all charges.

In the wake of the significant conviction, Lynette Woodrow from the Crown Prosecution Service emphasised the devastating physical and emotional repercussions of female genital mutilation, lasting a lifetime for the victims. Woodrow expressed empathy for the young girl, speculating on the immense pain and fear she likely experienced. Woodrow highlighted the vulnerability of a three-year-old, powerless to resist or defend herself, noting that the child had been coached to deceive the police but ultimately failed in doing so.

The Metropolitan Police revealed that initially, the victim had supported her parents' narrative in video-recorded interviews. However, she later provided a different account, stating that she had been restrained and subjected to cutting.

Both parents adamantly maintained their innocence and denied any role in the girl's mutilation throughout the investigation and trial. The mother's interest in witchcraft was discovered by the police during their investigation into the family. Findings of spells and curses at her home, including cow tongues bound with wire, nails, and a small knife in the freezer, were reported by the Crown Prosecution Services. Forty more limes and other fruits had pieces of paper inside with names on them.

After less than an hour of deliberation on Friday, the jury delivered a guilty verdict. The judge cautioned the tearful mother about an impending "lengthy" prison sentence, with a sentencing hearing scheduled for March 8.

Detective Chief Inspector Ian Baker emphasised the focus on the very young girl who fell victim to an illegal, horrific, and life-altering act at the hands of her mother.

b) Woman guilty of taking child to Kenya for mutilation

By Jeremy Britton

BBC News

Amina Noor, a 39-year-old woman from Harrow in north-west London, has been found guilty of transporting a three-year-old British child to Kenya for FGM. This marks the first conviction of aiding a non-UK person in performing FGM, and she is only the second person convicted of an FGM offence in England and Wales.

In 2006, Noor took the child to a private house for the procedure, claiming it was done for cultural reasons, citing her own experience as a child. Born in Somalia but holding British citizenship, Noor will be sentenced on December 20.

In 2015, the victim now 21, told a teacher about the FGM incident, which prompted the police to get involved. In 2019, a University College Hospital examination verified that the girl's clitoris had been completely removed.

During the trial, Noor asserted cultural pressure forced

her to comply. She claimed to have anticipated only a minor "touching" that would cause bleeding, not realising the extent of the mutilation.

The prosecution argued that Noor was aware FGM would be performed, whether it involved clitoral removal or other purposeless harm. Despite Noor denying threats, the prosecution emphasised her failure to inquire about the procedure or insist on her presence during it.

FGM is prevalent in the Somali community in East Africa, with UN figures indicating that 94% of Somali-origin women in Kenya have undergone this practice.

FGM AND THE NHS

The annual cost of providing NHS care for survivors of FGM is estimated to be £100 million. However, the current service provision by the NHS often falls short of optimal standards (5 Feb 2020).

For the treatment of FGM, specifically deinfibulation, surgery can be undertaken to open the vagina if necessary. The term "reversal," which is sometimes used to describe deinfibulation, is misleading because the procedure does not restore tissue that has been removed and cannot reverse the harm caused by FGM. However, it can deal with a number of issues brought on by FGM.

Surgery may be recommended for women facing challenges such as the inability to engage in sexual activity or difficulty urinating due to FGM. Pregnant women at risk of complications during labour or delivery as a result of FGM may also be advised to undergo deinfibulation. Ideally, the procedure should be performed before pregnancy. However, it can be done during pregnancy or labour if necessary, with the preference for completion before the last two months of pregnancy.

The deinfibulation surgery involves making an incision to open the scar tissue at the entrance to the vagina. Typically performed under local anaesthesia in a clinic, it usually does not require an overnight stay. In some cases, a small number of women may need a general anaesthetic or an epidural, which may entail a short hospital stay (NHS Overview).

National FGM Support Clinics (NFGMSCs) are community-based facilities providing various support services for women who have undergone FGM. Access to these services is free for individuals eligible for NHS care.

Scan below to visit the NHS webpage on FGM to find out more, and locate National Support Clinics.

SCAN ME

FGM-IS

Female Genital Mutilation - Information Sharing (FGM-IS) is a nationwide IT system designed to facilitate early intervention and continuous safeguarding for girls under the age of 18 with a familial background of FGM. This service enables authorised healthcare professionals and administrative personnel, including GPs, GP practice nurses, midwives, health visitors, school nurses, and local safeguarding leads across England, to access information pertaining to girls with a family history of FGM, irrespective of their care setting.

The FGM-IS streamlines the sharing of FGM-related data, eliminating organisations' need to duplicate information across systems. The service fosters national collaboration by offering real-time information from a centralised repository, all the while preserving data accuracy and minimising redundancy in information storage.

Advantages of the FGM-IS system include:

National Accessibility: Enables authorised healthcare

professionals across England to access information regarding girls with a family history of FGM, regardless of their location.

Information Dissemination: Facilitates the sharing of FGM-related information with authorised healthcare professionals and administrative staff who may come into contact with girls having a family history of FGM as they progress through life.

Safeguarding Enhancement: Offers an opportunity to reinforce local safeguarding frameworks and processes, contributing to the overall protection of at-risk individuals.

Compassionate Approach: Helps prevent the repeated questioning of girls and their families about the sensitive and potentially traumatic subject of FGM.

Examples of utilisation include:

- A General Practitioner utilising GP software is promptly notified about a family history of FGM during a consultation with a teenage girl, allowing for consideration of this information as a safeguarding concern.

- A midwife employing the National Childbirth and Reproduction System (NCRS) is alerted to a family history of FGM while consulting with a mother and her baby girl, providing an opportunity to discuss the matter as a safeguarding issue.

- A maternity nurse uses NCRS to document a family history of FGM for a newborn baby girl.

Additionally, a helpline (0800 028 3550) is available to support both professionals and family members who are concerned that a child is at risk of, or has undergone, FGM.

MEASURES AGAINST FGM

The implementation of a comprehensive strategy that incorporates legislative actions, educational initiatives, community engagement, and healthcare programmes can help nations combat FGM. It is insufficient to just make the practice illegal because it is not a cure-all. It is also essential not to perceive parents solely as criminals with harmful intent towards their daughters; rather, they may unknowingly participate in a criminal act.

Nevertheless, permitting a life-threatening practice to persist among innocent and defenceless children who cannot choose in the name of any customary law is unacceptable. Human life is of utmost value, and as civilised societies, we must protect it.

Countries can combat FGM through a combination of legal measures, education, community engagement, and healthcare initiatives.

Here are recommended actions for countries to address FGM:

1. **Legal Measures:**
   - Establish and enforce legislation explicitly prohibiting FGM, imposing stringent penalties to deter offenders.
   - Ensure the legal framework encompasses measures to prosecute those involved in performing or facilitating FGM.

Note that addressing customary practices through criminalisation and state repression may not eliminate them; rather, it may cause a reactionary response to maintain traditions. A more effective approach involves alternative methods, information networks, and targeted campaigns, particularly directed at parents. Responsibly informing parents about the serious risks associated with FGM is essential without criticising their perceptions.

2. **Education and Awareness:**
   - Conduct comprehensive public awareness campaigns to educate both urban and rural communities about the dangers and consequences of FGM.
   - Integrate information about FGM into school curricula to educate young people about the harmful impacts of the practice.
   - Engage religious and community leaders to advocate for the abandonment of FGM, given their significant influence in many societies.

3. **Community Engagement:**
   - Collaborate closely with local communities to instil a sense of ownership over the issue.

- Involve community leaders, elders, and women's groups in spreading the anti-FGM message.
- Establish safe spaces for open discussions challenging social norms surrounding the practice.

4. **Healthcare and Support Services:**
- Ensure access to medical and psychological support for females who have undergone FGM, addressing both physical and psychological complications.
- Provide training for healthcare providers to recognise and report cases of FGM, emphasising culturally sensitive care.

5. **International Cooperation:**
- Foster collaboration with international organisations, NGOs, and neighbouring countries to combat cross-border practices and support affected communities.

6. **Data Collection and Research:**
- Collect and analyse FGM prevalence and distribution data to tailor interventions and measure progress.
- Support research to understand the social, cultural, and economic factors contributing to FGM in specific regions.

7. **Alternative Rites of Passage:**
- Encourage the development and adoption of alternative rites of passage that preserve cultural traditions without resorting to FGM.

8. **Support Survivor Networks:**
- Promote the formation of networks and support groups for FGM survivors, offering emotional support, experience sharing, and advocacy against the practice.

9. **Monitoring and Evaluation:**
- Establish mechanisms to monitor the implementation and effectiveness of anti-FGM programs and policies.

10. **Long-term Planning:**

- Develop and implement long-term strategies to shift social norms and attitudes towards FGM, recognising that change may require sustained efforts over an extended period.

It is crucial to approach the issue of FGM with a holistic and culturally sensitive perspective, acknowledging local contexts and reasons behind the practice. Collaboration between government bodies, civil society, healthcare providers, and affected communities is essential for achieving lasting change.

The international community, including organisations like the United Nations (UN), is dedicated to ending FGM.

The United Nations takes a comprehensive approach to addressing FGM, involving various strategies:

1. **Resolutions and Declarations:** The UN General Assembly has consistently passed resolutions and declarations denouncing the practice of FGM. Member states are urged to implement measures to eradicate it. In 2012, for instance, a resolution specifically focused on eliminating FGM was adopted.
2. **UN Agencies:** Several UN agencies, including UNICEF (United Nations Children's Fund), UNFPA (United Nations Population Fund), and WHO (World Health Organization), actively engage in addressing FGM. They offer technical support, conduct research, and guide member states on strategies to tackle and prevent FGM.

3. **UNICEF's Focus:** UNICEF emphasises the importance of putting an end to FGM. UNICEF works in tandem with governments and civil society organisations to carry out awareness-raising initiatives, modify societal norms, and facilitate the passage of laws that forbid FGM.
4. **Sustainable Development Goals (SDGs):** The United Nations has integrated the elimination of FGM as a target under Goal 5 (Gender Equality) of the Sustainable Development Goals (SDGs). This underscores a global commitment to eradicating the practice by 2030.
5. **Data and Research:** UN organisations take an active role in gathering information and carrying out studies on the incidence and consequences of FGM. Precise information is necessary to assess the issue's extent and track advancement.
6. **Global Partnerships:** The UN collaborates with governments, non-governmental organisations, and other international bodies to establish a coordinated, global initiative against FGM.
7. **Advocacy and Awareness:** The UN plays a pivotal role in advocating for the abandonment of FGM and raising awareness about its detrimental effects.

The UN is working to end harmful practices, promote gender equality, and protect women's rights in addition to fighting FGM. Although there has been progress in many areas, FGM is still a deeply ingrained cultural practice in some, so the UN and its partners must continue to give this issue top priority.

The International Day of Zero Tolerance for FGM.

It was declared on February 6, 2003, by Stella Obasanjo, the First Lady of Nigeria and spokesperson for the Campaign Against Female Genital Mutilation. She made the official declaration during a conference organised by the Inter-African Committee on Traditional Practices Affecting the Health of Women and Children (IAC) in Africa. The purpose of this day, established by the UN, is to raise global awareness about the practice of FGM, which poses risks for women and brutally violates human rights.

Recently, the UNFPA-UNICEF Joint Programme on the Elimination of Female Genital Mutilation launched the 2023 theme, "Partnership with Men and Boys to Transform Social and Gender Norms to End FGM," as part of their ongoing efforts to eradicate this harmful practice.

7 Quotes About Female Genital Mutilation
By Joseph Osuigwe Chidiebere

"To cut off the sensitive sexual organ of a girl is directly against the honesty of nature, a distortion to her womanhood, and an abuse of her fundamental human right."

"The best way to make a girl to abstain from pre-marital sex is not by cutting her genital, but by educating and mentoring her"

"Together, we can build a nation where there is zero tolerance to female genital mutilation."

"Girls are well created, and it is unnecessary and irrelevant to cut any part of their bodies."

"You or any of your family members may not have practised female genital mutilation, but this is not enough reason to keep silent about it. You need to speak out against it to discourage others from the practice"

"When You circumcise a girl child, you affect her womanhood."

"Circumcisers make money from cutting girls/women, and girls/women (victims) spend money treating health complications of Female Genital Mutilation (AUGUST 6, 2017 Devatop Centre for Africa Development is a leading youth-led anti-human trafficking and human rights organisation in Nigeria)."

The African specialist **Nahid Toubia** puts it plain (when speaking of female genital mutilation): In a man, it would range from amputation of most of the penis to "removal of all the penis, its roots of soft tissue and part of the scrotal skin" (Eve Ensler, The Vagina Monologues).

Waris Dirie, in the Desert Flower, states: "These tribal wars, like the practice of circumcision, are brought about by the ego, selfishness, and aggression of men. I hate to say that, but it's true. Both acts stem from their obsession with their territory —their possessions—and women fall into that category both culturally and legally. Perhaps if we cut their balls off, my country would become a paradise. The men would calm down and be more sensitive to the world. Without that constant surge of testosterone, there'd be no war, no killing, no thieving, no rape. And if we chopped off their private parts and turned them loose to run around and either bleed to death or survive, maybe they could understand for the first time what they're doing to their women."

Some of the most famous activists in the fight against FGM are:

Ann-Marie Wilson

Dr. Ann-Marie Wilson was resolute in her belief that

additional efforts were essential to eliminate FGM, leading her to establish 28 Too Many. This UK-based organisation operates as an anti-FGM charity, extending its impact across 28 African countries while also prioritising collaboration with the diaspora in the UK.

"We often associate female genital mutilation with the horrific physical trauma... But there is less awareness about the psychological trauma that can haunt a woman throughout her lifetime."

Leyla Hussein

Leyla Hussein stands out as a prominent global advocate against FGM. Having personally survived FGM, she draws upon her own journey to develop effective social and political approaches to eliminate this harmful practice. Leveraging her background as a psychotherapist, Leyla emphasises the crucial necessity for increased psycho-social support for survivors. Notably, she co-founded the Dahlia Project and the non-profit organisation Daughter of Eve. Her recognition in German-speaking regions was significantly amplified through her involvement in the documentary "Female Pleasure."

"I might never be able to enjoy a sexual experience."

Mariya Karimjee

Mariya Karimjee courageously recounted her experience with FGM on a podcast episode of "This American Life." By shedding light on the often-overlooked problem of FGM in Pakistan, she has elevated the issue to public attention. As a survivor, Mariya has also openly discussed her journey towards reclaiming sexual pleasure, contributing to the crucial activism that breaks the silence surrounding the taboo subjects of sex and FGM. Her candid and honest approach works towards destigmatising these conversations, making them more accessible for broader societal discourse.

"This is child abuse, and they need to look at it as that. It is a child protection issue."

Hibo Wardere

Hibo Wardere, born in Somalia, is an advocate against FGM and the author of the enlightening biography titled "Cut: One Woman's Fight Against FGM in Britain Today." In her candid narrative of her personal encounter with FGM, Hibo highlights the fear and control imposed on young girls within practising communities.

"There is no authentic or relevant Islamic evidence allowing FGM in all its forms, and the practice is harmful and violates freedom, privacy, health and dignity of the Muslim woman."

Sheikh Ibrahim Lethome

Sheikh Ibrahim Lethome has devoted extensive efforts to dissociate FGM from Islam. Committing a significant portion of his life to the examination of pertinent religious texts, he has authored several publications that initiate religious dialogues on FGM and offer organisations strategies to detach the practice from Islam (Terri Harris, "5 Activists Fighting to End Female Genital Mutilation," Girls Globe, February 6, 2018).

However, this battle is substantial, and we recognise that the efforts of the UN and activists alone are insufficient. It requires organisations supported by volunteers and others to establish a comprehensive action plan in each region to effectively pursue the ultimate objective.

Many organisations are dedicated to fighting against FGM through advocacy, education, and support for affected communities. Here are 20 organisations that work to combat FGM:

1. The Desert Flower Foundation

The Desert Flower Foundation was founded in 2002 with the intention of permanently ending FGM by well-known model Waris Dirie and her partners. With 200 million girls impacted by the practice globally, the Foundation is committed to enlightening and educating people so they can actively prevent and rescue girls from FGM.

In the year of its inception, the Foundation conducted extensive research on FGM across Europe and Africa, culminating in a comprehensive 4,000-page report filled with factual information. This groundbreaking work prompted numerous governments and the European Union to prioritise FGM, including the issue on their agendas. Subsequently, legislative measures were implemented, and campaigns were initiated to combat this harmful practice.

At the moment, the Foundation is carrying out its worldwide campaigns to dissuade FGM and actively intervene to protect young girls in Africa. Through agreements with parents promising not to subject their daughters to FGM, the Foundation has been able to save thousands of girls. Additionally, it provides support to FGM survivors through healthcare, reconstructive surgery, and holistic hospital treatments. Furthermore, the Foundation is actively empowering women in Africa by offering education and training, enabling them to generate their own income.

2. **Equality Now**

It is an international entity dedicated to promoting a global environment where women and girls exercise autonomy over their bodies. Within the framework of Equality Now, FGM is viewed as a profound infringement of human rights intricately tied to gender equality and discrimination. The organisation actively advocates for the enactment of laws safeguarding girls. It lends support to local activists striving to eradicate FGM within their communities.

Equality Now works with regional partners, community mobilisation, and legal advocacy to push governments to enact laws that make FGM practices illegal. It encourages collaborations with people, organisations, and coalitions made up of corporations, women's organisations, activists, survivors, and legal reformers. Drawing upon their expertise and knowledge, the organisation endeavours to instigate transformative change. At the heart of their mission lies the provision of a platform for FGM survivors to voice their experiences and narratives, thereby fostering global awareness about this critical issue.

3. **ActionAid UK**

As a participant in ActionAid International, ActionAid UK is committed to collaborating with women and girls facing poverty. The organisation is devoted to eradicating violence against women and girls, aiming to transform their lives. Its efforts span three key areas: mobilising resources and generating funds through investments to combat poverty, advocating for change to confront violence and exploitation while striving for equal economic opportunities for women, and providing support during emergencies that jeopardise women's well-being.

The organisation actively engages in the fight against FGM in Ethiopia, Ghana, Kenya, Liberia, Senegal, Sierra Leone, Somalia, Gambia, and Uganda. Recognising that ending FGM requires a shift in societal attitudes and behaviours, the organisation offers assistance to women and girls who have escaped FGM through rescue centres, safe houses, and girls' clubs. In addition, it candidly discusses the negative impacts of FGM, actively working with nearby communities to educate them and empowering individuals to speak out and influence others on the issue through training programmes. The final objective is for every community to categorically reject FGM.

4. Wallace Global Fund

The Wallace Global Fund works to protect the diversity of nature and the vital natural systems that sustain all life by building an informed and involved citizenry. Eliminating FGM by 2030 is one of its main goals. In pursuit of this goal, the Fund collaborates with local communities, particularly in sub-Saharan Africa, Southeast Asia, and the Middle East, working closely with them to eliminate the practice.

A pivotal player in the Donors Working Group on FGM, the Fund collaborates with esteemed members such as UNFPA, UNICEF, USAID, the US State Department, and other multilateral and bilateral donors. Additionally, the Fund actively supports resource mobilisation endeavours and global advocacy initiatives. This support aims to ensure that advocates operating at the grassroots level receive both political backing and funding for their endeavours.

The Fund has also taken a proactive stance by sponsoring the Summit on Violence Against Girls and FGM in Washington, DC, which brought together over 200 activists and civil society organisations from across the globe. Furthermore, the Fund has championed the establishment of the US End FGM Network, designed to coordinate efforts among US groups dedicated to finding solutions to end and prevent FGM.

5. **28 Too Many**

Founded in 2010 in England and Wales, 28 Too Many is a charitable organisation dedicated to eradicating FGM in 28 African countries where the practice persists. At the grassroots level, the organisation gathers data and establishes community education and health networks. Its overarching mission is to catalyse a cascading impact that leads to the permanent cessation of FGM across Africa.

The organisation conducts extensive research and equips individuals and entities committed to ending FGM in African nations with knowledge and tools. With a vision of a world where every woman and girl is free from the threat of FGM, the organisation disseminates its collected data through various channels, such as country profile reports and thematic papers.

Making strategic use of the research findings, 28 Far too many actively engage influencers to promote change. It also creates advocacy materials that are given to neighbourhood organisations, enabling them to promote significant community change. Through these multifaceted efforts, the organisation strives to create a lasting positive impact, ultimately ending FGM in Africa.

6. Daughters of Eve

Daughters of Eve is a non-profit organisation dedicated to safeguarding young women and girls who face the threat of FGM. Its mission is to support and raise awareness for girls impacted by FGM, with the ultimate goal of eradicating this harmful practice.

According to the organisation, FGM is a type of gender-based violence that highlights the differences between men and women and puts the safety, security, autonomy, and well-being of its victims at risk. As a result, Daughters of is dedicated to protecting and advancing the rights of young people impacted by FGM in the areas where it is common in terms of their sexual, physical, mental, and reproductive health. The organisation takes a wholistic approach to healing and offers direction and help to enable and uplift these youth.

7. African Women Organization

Established in 1996, the African Women's Organization emerged as a non-governmental entity founded by women from diverse African nations such as Somalia, Ethiopia, Eritrea, Sudan, Nigeria, Senegal, Egypt, and others. Headquartered in Vienna, Austria, the organisation actively collaborates with various entities, including other organisations and government agencies, to address the challenges faced by immigrants and promote the welfare of women.

Since 1998, the organisation has prioritised its efforts towards combating FGM. Focusing on raising awareness, the organisation strives to eradicate this practice within immigrant communities whose members originate from countries at risk of FGM. Its activities include providing information and materials to students, researchers, and media outlets. In addition, the organisation creates kits for FGM training, trains trainers, provides consultation and advice to victims of FGM, and improves communication and cooperation with the FGM European network.

8. World Health Organization

Established in 1948, the World Health Organization (WHO) is a specialized agency of the United Nations dedicated to addressing global health concerns. The organisation's constitution, endorsed by 61 countries, marked its inception. Today, the WHO stands at the forefront of efforts to combat infectious diseases like HIV, Ebola, malaria, and tuberculosis. Beyond infectious diseases, the WHO also tackles issues related to sexual and reproductive health, nutrition, development, and food security.

The World Health Organisation actively combats FGM as one of its initiatives. In order to eradicate FGM, the World Health Assembly passed a resolution in 2008 highlighting the need for comprehensive action in a number of areas, including women's affairs, finance, education, and health. The WHO's approach involves providing training, policy, and guidelines to health professionals, empowering them to offer counselling and medical care to women and girls affected by FGM. Additionally, the organisation works towards building a robust evidence base by gathering information on the causes and consequences of FGM. Through advocacy efforts at international, regional, and local levels, the WHO strives to end the FGM practice.

9. End FGM European Network

The End FGM European Network (End FGM EU) constitutes a collaborative network comprising 24 European organisations in 13 countries across Europe. This collective effort is dedicated to eradicating FGM by fostering connections between communities and non-governmental organisations. The Network actively engages with all pertinent stakeholders addressing the FGM issue at both European and global levels.

End FGM EU is a central platform facilitating interaction and collaboration among organisations, European Union entities, and communities. Its function entails sharing knowledge and experiences in order to achieve the shared objective. The Network uses a number of tactics, such as gathering data, giving health programmes top priority, incorporating FGM into larger frameworks that address violence against women and girls, protecting refugees and asylum seekers who may be at risk of FGM, and advocating for the inclusion of FGM in EU global initiatives.

Since its establishment in 2009, the campaign to end FGM has garnered support from over 42,000 individuals who have endorsed the petition. Additionally, more than 50 members of the European Parliament have pledged their commitment to advocating for the inclusion of FGM in policies and legislation.

10. Safe Hands

Established in 2003 by Nancy Durrell McKenna, an acclaimed filmmaker and photographer, Safe Hands primarily aims to leverage the impact of photography and film to ensure the safety of every childbirth and pregnancy. The organisation functions around three main areas of competence. First, it works with service providers and community leaders to create messages that are appropriate and educate women and girls about relevant issues. Second, Safe Hands gives local community members the confidence to honestly express and tell their own stories. Last but not least, the group uses an evidence-based strategy to produce knowledge and create strong programmes that address the particular needs of women and girls.

In the realm of combating FGM, Safe Hands maintains a close collaboration with Hibo Wardere, a renowned anti-FGM campaigner. Wardere conducts training sessions for students, school administrations, and the police, equipping them with the skills to identify girls at risk of FGM and intervene effectively. Additionally, the organisation produces documentary films based on community storytelling to raise global awareness about the issue of FGM.

11. Beyond FGM

Beyond FGM envisions a world without genital mutilation and strives to achieve this through its mission. The organisation is dedicated to engaging with young girls, their families, and African midwives, fostering education and transforming perspectives on FGM. By collaborating with grassroots organisations, Beyond FGM aims to enhance their social change communications, contributing to eradicating FGM. The organisation builds partnerships with individuals, the African diaspora, and national entities, establishing a robust membership base involving young people, the media, corporations, and community leaders.

Drawing insights from the experiences of its members, Beyond FGM actively gathers knowledge on FGM. It advocates for the integration of FGM as a central component in the efforts of international organisations. It works towards securing increased commitments from donors to end FGM. The organisation's End FGM Grants Program supports explicitly grassroots organisations in Kenya, Nigeria, and the Gambia that are dedicated to ending FGM.

12. The UN Refugee Agency

The United Nations High Commissioner for Refugees is

the UN agency dedicated to safeguarding refugees, forcibly displaced individuals, and stateless people. The UNHCR not only gathers information on these vulnerable groups but also provides immediate assistance in the form of food, clean water, medical care, shelter, and other services. The group actively supports international efforts to eradicate FGM), runs awareness campaigns addressing the difficulties faced by refugees, and is instrumental in helping to relocate them to third countries.

The UNHCR is actively involved in combatting FGM among refugees placed in camps and certain urban areas, notably in countries like Yemen, Kenya, and Ethiopia. The organisation works to end FGM by offering safe havens to victims and addressing the health issues that women and girls face. It does this through awareness campaigns and community engagement projects. Additionally, the UNHCR gives them authority by promoting economic endeavours. The organisation works with governmental and civil society partners to protect and advocate for women and girls seeking refuge in the context of asylum seekers fleeing FGM.

13. FORWARD

FORWARD, the Foundation for Women's Health Research and Development stands at the forefront of African women-led initiatives dedicated to eradicating violence against women and girls. The organisation's comprehensive programs address the cessation of FGM, child marriage, and domestic and sexual violence. The overarching objective is to empower African women and girls, fostering a life of health and equality with dignity.

In the relentless battle against FGM, FORWARD collaborates closely with local communities, intervening to safeguard girls at risk of FGM and offering support to women affected by this harmful practice. Operating in Africa and among immigrant communities in the UK and Europe, the organisation actively engages with women and men. Through targeted initiatives, FORWARD offers training and activities to boost confidence while bringing attention to the dangers of FGM. This helps people advocate for radical change in their local communities, which advances the larger goals of eradicating FGM and advancing the welfare of women and girls.

14. The Girl Generation

The Girl Generation is an international African organisation that unites its members around the belief that FGM can and should be eliminated in this day and age. The Girl Generation is a force for social change because it offers a cohesive identity that opposes the cultural norms that support FGM. Through this platform, thousands of voices converge to advocate for abandoning FGM practices.

The organisation actively supports grassroots initiatives, tailoring efforts to address local contexts and enhancing social communications to combat FGM. By fostering partnerships with individuals, the African diaspora, and national organisations, and mobilising diverse groups including youth, media, community leaders, and corporations, The Girl Generation builds a formidable alliance against FGM.

Drawing on the extensive knowledge of its members, the organisation delves into local contexts. It gathers uplifting stories of social change from across the African continent and beyond, amplifying these narratives for widespread awareness. Additionally, The Girl Generation advocates for the integration of FGM eradication into international, regional, and national development policies.

In its commitment to supporting grassroots organisations with limited resources, The Girl Generation provides grants. Presently, these grants are accessible in Kenya, Nigeria, and the Gambia, empowering local efforts to end FGM.

15. Africa Coordinating Centre for the Abandonment of FGM/C

The Africa Coordination Centre for the Abandonment of

Female Genital Mutilation/Cutting (ACCAF) was founded in 2012 with the primary objective of addressing the existing gaps in efforts to eliminate FGM in the African region. The Centre's goals are to improve care for women and girls who suffer from the negative effects of FGM, as well as to strengthen research capacities and track developments in the abandonment of FGM.

Operating through a combination of community engagement and advocacy with governmental bodies, ACCAF works closely with communities affected by FGM. The organisation's programs empower women and girls by equipping them with skills and fostering confidence, enabling them to become advocates for change. ACCAF provides essential knowledge and tools to organisations involved with FGM-affected communities and conducts awareness campaigns to shed light on the issue. The organisation engages in advocacy efforts at various levels, ranging from grassroots organisations to government entities, to expedite the cessation of the practice.

Using its country, regional, and liaison offices network, ACCAF actively drives policy changes at all levels in the ongoing fight against FGM.

16.   Save the Children

Save the Children is one of the world's largest independent organisations dedicated to children, operating in approximately 120 countries. The organisation envisions a world where every child is entitled to protection, survival, development, and participation. Save the Children is committed to directly influencing global perspectives on children, striving for enduring positive transformations in their lives. Guided by core values such as accountability, ambition, collaboration, creativity, and integrity, the organisation engages in extensive efforts to combat harmful practices.

One significant focus is on preventing the prevalence of FGM in various countries. To empower women and girls to speak out against FGM in their communities and to educate them about the consequences of the practice, Save the Children organises educational workshops and get-togethers. The group also trains medical professionals so they can support those who have experienced FGM.

Save the Children adopts a comprehensive approach by offering support and alternative employment opportunities to those involved in carrying out FGM. This strategy aims to dissuade them from relying on such practices for their livelihoods. Furthermore, the organisation collaborates with religious leaders and youth groups, fostering awareness about the adverse effects of FGM. They disseminate knowledge within communities through creative mediums such as songs, poems, and plays, contributing to a broader understanding and rejection of FGM.

17. Orchid Project

The Orchid Project, a non-governmental organisation based in the UK, actively contributes to the global movement against FGM. Collaborating with grassroots organisations worldwide, the Orchid Project facilitates the exchange of knowledge to bring about meaningful change. The organisation also engages in advocacy efforts with governments, urging them to prioritise initiatives to eradicate FGM.

Currently, the Orchid Project works with community-based organisations in Mali, Kenya, Senegal, Gambia, Guinea, Guinea Bissau, and Guinea. In these areas, where FGM is ingrained in cultural customs, the Orchid Project highlights the importance of education grounded in human rights. One key tactic is to give communities the freedom to decide to stop FGM. By fostering connections between organisations and activists, the Orchid Project promotes sharing information and research, thereby catalysing global efforts to eliminate FGM.

The organisation's advocacy team plays a pivotal role in ensuring that the issue of FGM gains visibility on international platforms. They work closely with leaders and decision-makers to expedite actions and end the practice of FGM worldwide.

18. FGM National Clinical Group

The inception of the FGM National Clinical Group in 2007 marked a dedicated effort to support women impacted by FGM and associated concerns. The organisation is steadfast in its mission to enhance the well-being of women and their daughters exposed to the threat of FGM, leveraging research and clinical networks. Comprising healthcare professionals, advisors, and academics, the FGM National Clinical Group's collective goal is to eradicate the FGM practice. The organisation actively promotes the inclusion of FGM awareness in the training curricula for midwives, nurses, obstetricians, gynaecologists, and other healthcare professionals.

19. Plan International

Plan International is a humanitarian organisation dedicated to promoting children's rights and advancing gender equality, particularly for girls. The organisation collaborates with children, youth, and communities to identify and address the underlying causes of vulnerability and exclusion faced by girls. From birth through adulthood, Plan International supports children, equipping them to respond to crises and challenges. Utilising its knowledge and expertise, the organisation advocates for policy changes at various levels.

In the fight against FGM, Plan International works to change perceptions of the practice by interacting with parents, governments, children, and young people. In addition to spreading awareness about ending FGM, the organisation works to give girls the freedom to make decisions about their sexual and reproductive health. Plan International's fight against FGM places great emphasis on elevating the voices of young people and giving them the tools they need to actively participate in their rights advocacy and lead more satisfying lives.

20. Hope Foundation for African Women

The Hope Foundation for African Women (HFAW) is a global non-profit organisation dedicated to addressing gender inequalities in rural areas through initiatives focused on economic empowerment and promoting sexual and reproductive health. Central to HFAW's mission is its commitment to gender advocacy against FGM. To combat FGM, HFAW engages in dialogues with community leaders, with a special emphasis on religious leaders, recognising their influential role in shaping the views of their followers. HFAW prioritises outreach efforts in schools, religious institutions, markets, road shows, and the media to disseminate anti-FGM messages. Additionally, the organisation addresses broader issues such as children's rights, women's rights, and early pregnancies. Health promoters from HFAW conduct face-to-face discussions within communities, as highlighted in a feature by Human Rights Careers, "20 Organisations Fighting Female Genital Mutilation."

By raising awareness, providing support, and advocating for legislative changes targeted at eradicating FGM and defending the rights and welfare of women and girls, these organisations carry out essential tasks.

Here, I will cite the European Parliament resolution dated 12 February 2020 on the EU's strategy to eradicate FGM globally (2019/2988(RSP)).

The European Parliament,
— having regard to Articles 8 and 9 of Directive 2012/29/EU of the European Parliament and of the Council of 25 October 2012 establishing minimum standards on the rights, support and protection of victims of crime and replacing Council Framework Decision 2001/220/JHA ('the Victims' Rights Directive'), the provisions of which also apply to victims of female genital mutilation FGM,
— having regard to Articles 11 and 21 of Directive 2013/33/EU of the European Parliament and of the Council of 26 June 2013 laying down standards for the reception of applicants for international protection ('the Reception Conditions Directive'), which specifically mentions victims of FGM among the categories of vulnerable persons who should receive appropriate healthcare during their asylum procedures,
— having regard to Article 20 of Directive 2011/95/EU of the European Parliament and of the Council of 13 December 2011 on standards for the qualification of third-country nationals or stateless persons as beneficiaries of international protection for a uniform status for refugees or for persons eligible for subsidiary protection, and for the content of the protection granted ('the Qualification Directive'), in which FGM as a serious form of psychological, physical or sexual violence is included as a ground to be taken into consideration for granting international protection,
— having regard to its resolution of 14 June 2012 on ending female genital mutilation, which called for an end to FGM worldwide through prevention, protection measures and legislation,

— having regard to its resolution of 6 February 2014 on the Commission communication entitled 'Towards the elimination of female genital mutilation',
— having regard to its resolution of 7 February 2018 on zero tolerance for FGM,
— having regard to the EU Annual Reports on Human Rights and Democracy in the World, in particular its resolution of 15 January 2020,
— having regard to the Council conclusions of June 2014 on preventing and combating all forms of violence against women and girls, including female genital mutilation,
— having regard to the Council conclusions of 8 March 2010 on the eradication of violence against women in the European Union,
— having regard to the Commission communication of 25 November 2013 entitled 'Towards the elimination of female genital mutilation' (COM(2013)0833),
— having regard to the joint statement of 6 February 2013 on the International Day against Female Genital Mutilation, in which the Vice-President of the Commission / High Representative of the Union for Foreign Affairs and Security Policy and five Commissioners reaffirmed the EU's commitment to combating FGM in its external relations,
— having regard to the EU Action Plan on Human Rights and Democracy 2015-2019, in particular Objective 14(b), which specifically mentions FGM, and taking into consideration the Action Plan's current revision and the negotiations for its renewal,
— having regard to the experience acquired through implementing the Commission's Strategic Engagement for Gender Equality 2016-2019 and through pursuing the measures set out in the action plan forming part of the Commission's communication of 25 November 2013,
— having regard to the 2030 Agenda for Sustainable

Development, in particular Target 5.3 on eliminating all harmful practices, such as child, early and forced marriage and female genital mutilation,

— having regard to the 1994 International Conference on Population and Development (ICPD) in Cairo and its Programme of Action, and to the outcomes of subsequent review conferences, in particular the Nairobi Summit on ICPD25, and its commitment to zero FGM,

— having regard to the Beijing Platform for Action and the outcomes of its subsequent review conferences,

— having regard to the Gender Action Plan 2016-2020 (GAP II), in particular its Thematic Priority B, which has a specific indicator on FGM, and taking into consideration its current revision and the negotiations for its renewal,

— having regard to the commitment by the President of the Commission to adopting measures to tackle violence against women, as stated in her Political Guidelines,

— having regard to the anticipated new EU Gender Equality Strategy,

— having regard to the European Institute for Gender Equality (EIGE) report of 2013 on 'Female genital mutilation in the European Union and Croatia', as well as the two subsequent reports entitled 'Estimation of girls at risk of female genital mutilation in the European Union' of 2015 on Ireland, Portugal and Sweden, and of 2018 on Belgium, Greece, France, Italy, Cyprus and Malta,

— having regard to the Council of Europe Convention on preventing and combating violence against women and domestic violence ('the Istanbul Convention') of 2014, Article 38 of which requires the criminalisation of FGM by all state parties,

— having regard to its resolution of 12 September 2017 on the proposal for a Council decision on the conclusion by the European Union of the Council of Europe Convention

on preventing and combating violence against women and domestic violence (COM(2016)0109 — 2016/0062(NLE)),
— having regard to its resolution of 28 November 2019 on the EU's accession to the Istanbul Convention and other measures to combat gender-based violence,
— having regard to the Declaration of the Council of Europe Committee of Ministers of 13 September 2017 on the need to intensify the efforts to prevent and combat female genital mutilation and forced marriage in Europe,
— having regard to the WHO guidelines on the management of health complications from female genital mutilation,
— having regard to the UN Human Rights Council resolution of 5 July 2018 on the 'Elimination of female genital mutilation',
— having regard to the United Nations Secretary-General report of 27 July 2018 on 'Intensifying global efforts for the elimination of female genital mutilation',
— having regard to the UN General Assembly resolution of 14 November 2018 on 'Intensifying global efforts for the elimination of female genital mutilation',
— having regard to the Cotonou Agreement and its ongoing revision process,
— having regard to the EU-UN Spotlight Initiative of September 2017 on eliminating violence against women and girls,
— having regard to Rule 132(2) of its Rules of Procedure,

A. whereas FGM is considered internationally to constitute a gross and systematic violation of human rights, a form of violence against women and girls and a manifestation of gender inequality, not connected to any one religion or culture, and is now recognised as a global issue affecting at least 200 million women and girls in 30 countries, according to statistical reports from UNICEF, the UNFPA and the WHO; whereas, however, there is evidence of the occurrence of FGM in over 90 countries across all continents;

B. whereas, according to 2018 UNFPA data, if population trends continue in the direction they are currently moving in, 68 million girls worldwide will be at risk of FGM by 2030, with the yearly increase expected to rise from an estimated 4,1 million in 2019 to 4,6 million per year by 2030;

C. whereas, according to the most recent national data available across Europe, it is estimated that around 600 000 women and girls in Europe are living with the lifelong physical and psychological consequences of FGM, and a further 180 000 girls are at a high risk of FGM in 13 European countries alone;

D. whereas FGM comprises all procedures that involve partial or total removal of the external female genitalia, such as clitoridectomy, excision, infibulation and other harmful procedures, and that intentionally alter or cause injury to the female genital organs for non-medical purposes, producing physical, sexual, and psychological health complications that can lead to death;

E. whereas FGM is mostly carried out on young girls between infancy and the age of 15 whereas. Moreover, a girl or woman can be subjected to FGM on multiple occasions throughout her life, for example, when she is imminently about to be married or when she is about to depart on a trip abroad;

F. whereas, a recent increase in the percentage of women and girls potentially already affected by FGM, according to 2018 data from the Office of the UNHCR, means that the relevance of the issue is becoming even greater and the number of those affected or at risk is continuing to grow; whereas, according to the UNHCR, over 100 000 female asylum seekers potentially affected by FGM arrived in Europe in the last five years alone;

G. whereas, according to UNICEF, progress has been

achieved with the risk of FGM for girls being one-third less today than it was 30 years ago. However, taking into account all the available data, and with 10 years to go until 2030, Sustainable Development Goal 5.3 on the elimination of FGM is far from being achieved; whereas the absolute numbers of women and girls affected appear, on the contrary, to be on the increase and continue to increase unless massively scaled-up efforts are urgently taken to prevent this from happening;

H. whereas, to accelerate change and achieve the goal of ending FGM worldwide by 2030, there is an urgent need to scale up and coordinate existing efforts to end the practice at local, national, regional and international levels to capitalise on these efforts and bring about increased and lasting change through effective and comprehensive strategies;

I. whereas FGM is a form of gender-based violence and addressing the root causes of gender inequality at the community level, including gender stereotypes and harmful social norms, is essential to put an end to FGM;

J. whereas FGM is often indissociable from other gender inequality issues and is but one of many violations of women's rights, such as the lack of access to education for girls, including comprehensive sexual education, the lack of employment for women, the inability to own or inherit property, forced or early child marriage, sexual and physical violence, and the lack of quality healthcare, including sexual and reproductive health and rights services;

K. whereas the 'medicalisation' of FGM is the practice of FGM carried out by a healthcare professional or in a hospital or medical facility; whereas the medicalisation of FGM is a dangerous attempt to legitimise the practice of FGM and even potentially to profit from it;

1. Reiterates its commitment to help eliminate the practice of FGM worldwide as a form of gender-based violence that has long-lasting psychological and physical consequences on women and girls and, in some instances, causes death;
2. Notes that the recognition of The Restorers on the shortlist for the Sakharov Prize marks an important step in this direction and in the fight against FGM; further recognises the important role of young people in empowering themselves and others by becoming role models within their own communities;
3. Stresses that the primary goal of any action relating to FGM must be its prevention through sustainable societal change and the empowerment of communities, and specifically of the women and girls within them, through the provision of education and information and by creating the preconditions for the economic empowerment of women and girls; underlines that the protection and aftercare of survivors of FGM must be a priority to be achieved by providing adequate protection and information, and access to professional and adequate physical, psychological, medical and sexological care and support for survivors of this practice through increased investment;
4. Underlines that the involvement of men and boys in the process of reshaping gender relations and changing behaviour and in supporting the empowerment of women and girls is equally crucial to the elimination of this harmful practice; stresses, furthermore, the importance of involving community leaders in ending FGM,

as it is transmitted through traditions and culture, using cutters and circumcisers, who often have influential roles within communities, and using diverse religions as legitimation for carrying out and passing on this practice;

5. Stresses that FGM must be tackled through a holistic and intersectional approach, addressing the root causes of gender inequality that underlie all forms of gender-based violence against all women and girls, including violations of their human rights, physical integrity and sexual and reproductive health and rights, and, in particular, linking FGM to other harmful practices such as early and forced marriage, breast ironing, hymenoplasty and virginity testing;

6. Is worried about the increasingly widespread phenomenon of the 'medicalisation' of FGM in some countries — even those in which FGM is illegal — and the growing involvement of health professionals in this practice; insists that this is an unacceptable response in addressing the root causes of FGM, as has already been established by the UN and the WHO; invites the countries concerned to explicitly outlaw the medicalisation of FGM while raising awareness among medical staff about this problem through the provision of information and training, as well as adequate supervision and enforcement;

7. Underlines that, under Article 38 of the Istanbul Convention, the Member States are under an obligation to criminalise FGM, as well as the incitement, coercion or procurement of a girl to undergo it, and that the Convention protects not only girls and women at risk from FGM, but also girls and women who are suffering the lifelong consequences of this practice; is pleased to note

that criminal law in all Member States protects girls and women from FGM, but is extremely concerned about its apparent ineffectiveness, with only a handful of cases reaching court in the EU;

8. Notes that in many EU countries, it is also possible to prosecute FGM performed abroad, per the principle of extra-territoriality, which therefore also prohibits the taking of children to third countries to undergo FGM; notes that criminalisation must be matched with prosecutions and investigations; stresses that the best interests of the child must always be a primary consideration, and that the process of prosecuting and convicting family members who carry out FGM practices must also ensure that the girls and children involved are not put at further risk as a consequence;

9. Calls on the Commission and the Member States to ensure that the future EU budget, both internally and externally, continues to support the sustainability of community engagement in projects and programmes through adequate funding that takes into account the operational realities of community-based organisations and survivor-and youth-led organisations and initiatives; to this end, calls on the Commission and the Council to ensure the flexibility, accessibility and sustainability of funding based on structural financial support in the longer term within the budgetary discussions on the next multiannual financial framework (MFF);

10. Welcomes the work already accomplished through the Rights, Equality and Citizenship Programme and calls on the Commission and the Member States to ensure that the future EU budget

takes the need for greater flexibility and for synergies between internal and external funding programmes into account, to promote budgets which address the complexity of the issue, as well as more comprehensive transnational and cross-border interventions to achieve the global eradication of FGM;

11. Encourages the Commission and the Member States to strengthen their engagement with European and national networks of professionals, including those in the areas of health, social care, law enforcement and civil society, and to ensure that EU funding goes to projects aimed at training and awareness-raising campaigns for professionals on how to effectively prevent, detect and respond to cases of FGM and violence against women and girls;

12. Urges the Commission to ensure that all Member States translate the 'Victims' Rights Directive' into national legislation and fully implement it to ensure that the survivors of FGM can access confidential specialist support services, including trauma support and counselling, as well as shelters, in emergency situations in the EU;

13. Notes that access to specialist healthcare, including psychological care, for female asylum seekers and refugees who are survivors of FGM must be considered as a priority at both EU and Member State levels, in the light of the latest UNHCR data;

14. Calls on the Commission and the Council to ensure that within the reform of the Common European Asylum System (CEAS), the highest international protection standards on qualification, reception conditions and

procedural rights are applied homogenously across the EU, facilitating strong cooperation between the Member States, particularly concerning vulnerable female asylum seekers affected by or at risk of FGM and other forms of gender-based violence;

15. Urges the Commission, in the light of the increase in the number of women and girls affected by FGM, to launch a review of the 2013 communication entitled 'Towards the elimination of female genital mutilation' in order to ensure the scaling up of actions against the practice worldwide, and that work is done to tackle the disparities in laws, policies and service provision between the Member States so that women and girls affected or at risk of FGM can access equal standards of treatment throughout the EU;

16. Calls on the Commission to ensure that the forthcoming Gender Equality Strategy includes actions to end FGM and to provide care for survivors, that it contains inclusive language, strong commitments and clear indicators in all areas of EU competence, together with regular reporting and a strong monitoring mechanism, so that it ensures the accountability of all EU institutions and Member States;

17. Calls on the Commission, the European External Action Service (EEAS) and the Member States to step up cooperation with third countries in order to encourage them to adopt national laws banning FGM, to support law enforcement authorities in ensuring the implementation of these laws and to prioritise the issue of FGM and other practices harmful to women and girls in its external human rights policy,

notably in its bilateral and multilateral human rights dialogues and other forms of diplomatic engagement; stresses that the EU can help to eradicate FGM around the world by establishing and encouraging best practices here in the EU;

18. Calls on the Commission to ensure that the forthcoming Gender Action Plan III continues to include among its pivotal actions the eradication of FGM and the provision of care for survivors as part of the fight against all forms of violence against women and girls through concrete and trackable indicators;

19. Calls on the Commission, including the EEAS, to ensure that the forthcoming new EU Action Plan on Human Rights and Democracy continues to include among its objectives the eradication of FGM and the provision of care for survivors;

20. Reiterates its call on the Council to urgently conclude the EU ratification of the Istanbul Convention based on a broad accession without any limitations and to advocate its ratification by all the Member States; calls on the Council and the Commission to ensure the full integration of the Convention into the EU legislative and policy framework to ensure the prevention of FGM, protection of women and prosecution of offenders and adequate provision of services in response to FGM by all State Parties;

21. Reiterates its calls on the Commission and the Member States to mainstream the prevention of FGM in all sectors, especially in health, including sexual and reproductive health and rights, social work, asylum, education, including sexual education, employment, law enforcement, justice, child protection, media, technology and communication; calls for the establishment

of multi-stakeholder platforms between the different sectors to better coordinate such cooperation;

22. Welcomes the Commission's efforts and its active promotion of the elimination of FGM through internal discussions with civil society and external policies through dialogues with partner countries, as well as its commitment to a yearly assessment of the EU's fight against FGM;

23. Calls on the Commission and the Member States to ensure that appropriate and structured mechanisms are in place to meaningfully engage with FGM-affected community representatives and grassroots women's organisations, including survivor-led organisations, in policy and decision-making;

24. Calls on the Commission to ensure, through the inclusion of human rights clauses, that EU cooperation and trade agreements with third countries are negotiated and reviewed in line with their compliance with international human rights standards, including the elimination of FGM as a systematic human rights violation and a form of violence hindering the full development of women and girls;

25. Welcomes the updated methodology contained in the 'Estimation of girls at risk of female genital mutilation in the European Union: Step-by-step guide (2nd edition)' published by the EIGE and aimed at gathering more accurate and robust data; calls on the Commission and the Member States to update the relevant data and address the lack of reliable, comparable statistics at EU level on the prevalence of FGM and its types, and to involve academics, as well as practising communities and survivors, in the

process of data collection and research, through a community-based and participatory approach; urges organisations, governments, and the EU institutions to work together to provide more accurate qualitative and quantitative information on FGM, and to make it available and accessible to the wider public; encourages, furthermore, the exchange of best practices and cooperation among the relevant authorities (police and prosecutors), including international alerts;
26. Calls on the Commission to invest more sustainable funds in research into FGM, as producing in-depth qualitative and quantitative research is the only way to promote a better understanding of the phenomenon and ensure it is targeted in a tailored and effective way;
27. Instructs its President to forward this resolution to the Commission and the Council.

In conclusion, FGM is a deeply entrenched practice with serious physical and psychological consequences. A combination of legislative action, community engagement, education, and cultural sensitivity must be used in the fight to eradicate it. Even though there has been an increase in awareness and a decrease in the frequency of FGM, more work needs to be done globally to guarantee the rights and welfare of girls and women everywhere and to bring an end to this harmful practice.

"A culture where Nature has become the exception is a culture in trouble"

GABOR MATE, "The Myth of Normal"

PART THREE

Menstrual Hygiene Day, also called Period Day, is observed on May 28. Today is a chance to confront the social stigmas associated with menstruation, which frequently have a negative impact on those who go through them. People have been wearing period bracelets on this day for many years in an effort to raise awareness of menstrual concerns. These bracelets serve as a straightforward educational tool, featuring five red beads representing the days of bleeding and other beads signifying the remainder of the menstrual cycle. They have evolved into a symbol emphasising that menstruation cannot be concealed (Wateraid, 2021).

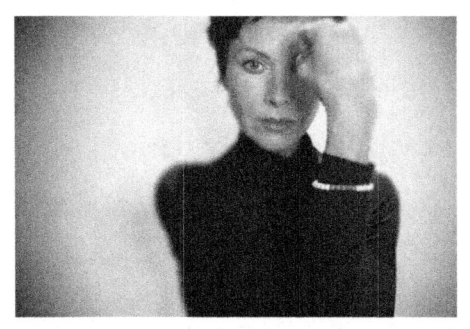

Period bracelet in white and red (Wateraid, 2021).

Approximately 1.8 billion individuals experience menstruation every month globally, equating to 800 million women and girls menstruating at any given time. This is 26% of the global population, and a lot of people feel ashamed about the experience. An estimated 500 million people do not have access to adequate facilities for managing menstrual hygiene or menstrual products.

UNESCO reports that only 50% of Kenyan girls can access sanitary pads. In Nepal and Afghanistan, 30% of girls miss school during menstruation, while in India, 20% drop out entirely. The affordability of menstrual products varies across countries, with the least affordable being Algeria (14.8%), Zambia (10.93%), Nigeria (10.93%), Ghana (9.39%), Zimbabwe (9.27%), Kyrgyzstan (9.05%), Honduras (8.54%), Jordan (8.38%), Laos (8.33%), and Cambodia (7.74%).

One in eight women in the UK didn't know about periods until they started having menstruation. Furthermore, a troubling proportion of people hold onto myths, such as the notion that one shouldn't exercise or that one cannot become pregnant while on their period. Approximately one-third of women are uncomfortable talking to others about their menstrual cycle. These misconceptions and societal norms surrounding menstruation are prevalent worldwide, as highlighted in the article "Why we shouldn't be ashamed of being PeriodProud," published on May 25, 2018, by Hannah Jarratt of WaterAid.

"The most common misconception I hear from my patients is that a period is a healthy way for the body to "cleanse" itself every month. This sounds lovely, in theory, but is false", says **Maria Sophocles**, *M.D., a board-certified ob-gyn and the medical director of Women's Healthcare of Princeton.*

"Sharks are certainly attracted to blood but there is a 9:1

ratio of males to females in terms of shark attacks, so the fact that you are on your period is likely irrelevant", says Dr Sophocles.

"There's no reason to adjust your workout during your cycle except if you bleed very heavy and feel more fatigued", says **Alyse Kelly-Jones**, M.D., a board-certified ob-gyn with Novant Health Mintview in Charlotte, North Carolina.

6 of the most common period myths:

Myth 1:

The belief that menstrual blood is impure and filled with toxins is entirely unfounded. Contrary to misconceptions, menstrual blood does not detoxify the body. While it differs from the blood circulating in our veins regarding concentration and red blood cell count, this disparity doesn't imply any abnormal conditions in the sensitive area.

Myth 2:

The idea that one cannot become pregnant by engaging in sexual activity during menstruation falls under both contraception and period-related myths. For women with irregular or shorter cycles or those experiencing heavier bleeding, there's a potential overlap between the fertile window and the menstrual period. It's advised not to take risks based on this misconception.

Myth 3:

The notion that one should avoid bathing during menstruation is rooted in myths that suggest water either promotes or halts bleeding. It's crucial to clarify that immersing oneself in a tub doesn't halt bleeding; it merely temporarily stems from the flow due to water pressure. Warm water, especially in heavy bleeding cases, can alleviate cramps and reduce muscle tension.

Myth 4:

The belief that women lose so much blood during menstruation that they might faint is exaggerated. The actual amount of blood lost during a period is around 30-40 ml, equivalent to 2 to 3 tablespoons. For most women, this is not a cause for concern. However, if someone experiences menorrhagia (excessive bleeding), it is advisable to consult a doctor.

Myth 5:

Contrary to the misconception that exercising during menstruation is harmful, physical activity can be beneficial. Even in gentle activities like walking or swimming, exercise is a friend to those dealing with menstrual cramps. While extreme activities may not be necessary, moderate exercise can alleviate discomfort and enhance mood.

Myth 6:

The idea that women's menstrual cycles synchronise when spending much time together lacks scientific support. Despite some low-quality studies, no mechanism has been proposed to explain this phenomenon. Instances where periods seemingly align with those of others are often attributed to selective memory, specifically the tendency to remember synchronised cycles while overlooking instances when they do not occur (confirmation bias).

Strange myths about the period exist in different countries of the world:

ARGENTINA If you try to make whipped cream, it will turn sour.

BRAZIL Walking barefoot during your period will cause cramps.

FRANCE Mayonnaise you make while on your period will cut through.

USA/CANADA You shouldn't go camping because bears can smell the period from afar.

JAPAN Your sense of taste is not right, avoid making sushi.

INDIA Girls believe they can't touch, or share food, or hug family members when they are on their period.

ITALY You should avoid swimming in the sea or the pool.

COLOMBIA When you have your period, you should avoid cold drinks because they will give you cramps.

MEXICO Dancing during period damages the uterus.

POLAND Sex during your period can kill your partner.

ROMANIA Don't touch the flowers when you have your period because they will wither faster.

MADAGASCAR Menstruating Malagasy women are told not to use the front door

NIGERIA It can even be taboo to hold your baby at that time of the month.

NEPAL According to the funniest legend: It's thought that people on their period shouldn't touch animals, while at the same time, in Nepal, the practice of Chhaupadi is applied even nowadays.

MENSTRUAL TABOOS

Cultural, social, and historical taboos surrounding menstruation have persisted for centuries despite it being a normal and essential biological process that most females go through. Even with the recent progress made in breaking the taboo around menstruation, there are still many parts of the world where this topic is still stigmatised.

Historical Backdrops of Menstruation Taboos Throughout history, menstruation has been veiled in myths, superstitions, and taboos. Many societies deemed menstruating women impure, associating their touch or presence with bad luck. These beliefs often resulted in isolation and exclusion, with women segregated during their periods. These taboos possess deep-seated roots, perpetuated through generations.

Influence of Religion and Culture The taboo nature of menstruation has been cemented in large part by cultural and religious beliefs. It has been interpreted in some cultures that menstruation is dirty or impure, which has led to the stigmatisation of menstruation and prevented open communication. Christianity, Judaism, Islam, Buddhism, and Hinduism have all portrayed menstruation negatively, imposing restrictions on menstruators, such as barring entry to Eastern Orthodox churches or participation in communion. Shintos are prohibited from visiting temples or ascending sacred mountains during menstruation in Japan.

Social Stigma and Gender Disparity Menstruation taboos have perpetuated gender inequality by reinforcing stereotypes and constraining opportunities for girls and women. The societal imposition of shame and a sense of uncleanness during periods often result in diminished self-esteem and self-worth for women and girls. Additionally, the lack of access to menstrual hygiene products and secure, private facilities for managing menstruation exacerbates challenges faced by women in various parts of the world.

Addressing Menstrual Taboos: A Shift in Perspectives

In recent years, a global movement has emerged, actively challenging and dismantling the long-standing taboos surrounding menstruation. This transformative shift is attributed to several key factors:

1. **Educational Initiatives:** A pivotal step in breaking the menstruation taboo involves comprehensive education. By imparting knowledge about

the biological processes and emphasising the significance of menstruation, individuals are less likely to perpetuate stigmatising beliefs.
2. **Advocacy and Awareness Campaigns:** There are a lot of people and groups working to increase public awareness of menstruation and related issues. Menstrual health is tirelessly promoted by events like Menstrual Hygiene Day, which also contributes to the continuous effort to break taboos.
3. **Enhanced Access to Menstrual Hygiene Products:** Endeavors are underway to ensure affordable and safe menstrual hygiene products are readily available to women and girls. This not only upholds dignity but also challenges the notion that menstruation should be concealed or met with shame.
4. **Challenge to Cultural and Religious Beliefs:** A burgeoning movement is contesting how cultural and religious texts are interpreted in ways that support the stigma associated with menstruation. Activists and scholars are actively presenting alternative, inclusive, and empowering perspectives.
5. **Education for Boys:** Dr Fabian Almeida, a Consultant Psychiatrist at Fortis Hospital, Kalyan, emphasises the importance of educating boys about menstruation: "A man who knows that menstruation is the most scientific process the human body can face will show empathy towards a woman during her menstrual cycle". Providing detailed information about the menstrual cycle helps boys understand that menstruation is a natural and scientific process. This knowledge fosters empathy and encourages open discussions, discouraging inappropriate jokes at the expense of girls.

Boys should be educated about menstruation at home and school to ensure genuine awareness. By explaining the meaning of various expressions related to menstruation, such as "I'm not in the mood" or "the Russians have come", and using positive terminology, boys can be empowered to engage in respectful conversations about a topic that affects half of the world's population every month. There is no reason why they shouldn't learn about this essential aspect of human biology.

"When Sally Ride went into space (the first American woman to do so), scientists in NASA asked her if 100 tampons would be enough for a week. That's right. 100! Let's make menstruation a part of men's regular lives too" (How to Talk About Your Period With Men Post author: Martha Michaud, Post published: September 23, 2020).

The "Pad Man"

He pioneered an affordable sanitary napkin that shattered the period taboo in conservative India, where just 10% of women reportedly utilised such products.

Arunachalam Muruganantham, newly married, discovered his wife concealing a soiled cloth—one he deemed unfit even for his motorcycle. Purchasing sanitary napkins for her, he encountered a store clerk discreetly wrapping the package in a newspaper. He recognised the cotton-based product's simplicity and cost-effectiveness and envisioned a similar solution.

Despite facing challenges, including persuading volunteers to test his prototypes, only his wife initially offered assistance. However, she eventually withdrew her support, suspecting ulterior motives. Seeking help from medical students, he encountered reluctance but persevered in testing the products himself to assess usability.

His wife and he separated as a result of worsening personal and financial issues. Unfazed, he succeeded in creating a reasonably priced sanitary pad manufacturing machine by 2000. Upon realising his success, his wife came back to help him fulfil his mission.

He manufactured numerous sanitary pads with a simple yet effective machine, distributing them to rural areas where economically disadvantaged women resided. He became a catalyst for change in a country where many used leaves, barks, or even sawdust during menstruation.

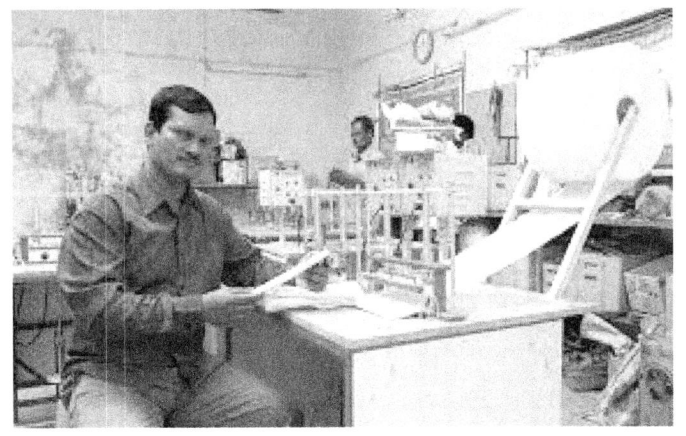

"The Pad Man", Arunachalam Muruganantham (Baral, 2018)

Despite a school dropout background, he transformed conservative India, supplying sanitary pads to 4,500 Indian villages and 19 countries. His aspiration is to make sanitary pads ubiquitous for all Indian women.

TIME magazine recognised his impact, listing him among the world's most powerful people in 2014, and in 2016, he received India's highest civilian honour, the "Padma Shri."

Be Girl

Diana Sierra, a Colombian social entrepreneur and industrial designer, serves as the co-founder and CEO of Be Girl, as mentioned in a Columbia University Earth Institute article dated September 21, 2021.

In 2012, during her work in Uganda, Diana Sierra

witnessed girls dropping out of school due to a lack of resources for managing their periods. Upon delving deeper into the issue, she realised that while items like books and shoes were essential, addressing the fundamental challenge of gender neglect was crucial. It became evident that without tackling this issue, gender inequality would persist, infiltrating various aspects of a girl's life from the classroom to adulthood.

Working closely with the affected girls, Sierra discovered that the problem extended beyond access to traditional sanitary supplies. There was a need for a solution tailored to their bodies, cultural practices, and available resources. Through multiple prototype iterations, the signature colourful, hybrid design with a waterproof bottom and mesh pocket emerged, tested and improved with the girls. Diana recognised the revolutionary impact of the product when one girl enthusiastically exclaimed, "What I like best -- it makes me proud to be a girl!"

Be Girl is a social enterprise that was established in 2014 and is motivated by the idea that every girl deserves to feel proud of herself on every day of the month. The organisation is dedicated to meeting the needs of the more than 250 million teenage girls who do not have access to menstruation products that are appropriate and perform well. Be Girl seeks to advance self-reliance and female emancipation while maintaining a sustainable environmental impact.

Zana Africa-Nia

In 2007, **Megan White Mukuria** founded ZanaAfrica after discovering, while working with Kenyan children in 2001, that 65% of girls lacked access to sanitary pads and essential health education to navigate the challenges of growing up. Headquartered in Nairobi, Kenya, with a US subsidiary, ZanaAfrica produces eco-friendly pads in Kenya. The organisation initially introduced two lines of sanitary pads: Safi pads for purchase and Nia pads distributed free to girls through local organisations. However, as of 2020, only Nia pads appear to be available for purchase.

ZanaAfrica envisions a world where girls and women in East Africa lead healthy, safe, and educated lives while defining their own purpose. They advocate for menstrual health management as a human right, emphasising puberty as an ideal time to engage girls in various personal health decisions. The ZanaAfrica Group aims to provide dignity and inspire women and girls to fulfil their purpose through sanitary pads and related products.

Several other organisations work to guarantee that hygiene products are available to women and girls throughout Africa, in addition to ZanaAfrica. It is important to recognise that, according to data from WaterAid, 1.25 billion women worldwide do not have access to a toilet during their menstrual cycle.

Another notable initiative is led by Indian-born author **Aditi Gupta**, who created **Menstrupedia**, a comic addressing menstruation taboos in India in a lighthearted manner. The comic's goal is to help girls in India understand menstruation and maintain health and activity during their periods and throughout their lives. Similar initiatives exist in countries like Kenya, Indonesia, Madagascar, and beyond, demonstrating a global commitment to menstrual equity.

Scan below to visit the Menstrupedia webpage and view the work they do, find out about their latest projects, and even purchase the Menstrupedia comic.

ACTIVISTS AND AMNESTY INTERNATIONAL

At this point, I quote the experiences of 5 activists who broke the taboos surrounding menstruation that came to light thanks to Amnesty International.

Zhanar Sekerbayeva, aged 36, serves as an LBQ activist and is the founder of Feminita, an initiative dedicated to advocating for feminism and safeguarding the rights of lesbian, bisexual, and queer women in Kazakhstan.

In Kazakhstan, discussing menstruation openly remains a challenge. Instead, individuals resort to euphemisms like Red Aunty, Red October, or Red Army. When I experienced my first period, my mother, a paediatrician, handed me a piece of cloth without providing any explanation of its purpose or usage. If a girl experiences a period leak at school, it becomes a subject of mockery, and teachers may send her home. Some resort to burying their stained panties or using unhygienic materials, leading to reproductive health issues.

Seeing the need for change, I took part in a photo shoot

addressing the taboos surrounding menstruation in Almaty, Kazakhstan, along with a group of nonviolent protestors. With our hand-drawn posters that included images and slogans, we set out to question accepted social mores. Following the demonstration, I found myself confronted by seven policemen as I exited a café. They demanded I accompany them to the station, threatening physical force if I refused.

I faced charges of minor hooliganism and underwent extensive questioning by a judge. The interrogation delved into the content of the poster I held, accompanied by intrusive personal inquiries like my marital status, motherhood, and pregnancy. I asserted my identity as an openly lesbian individual, redirecting the focus to my partner instead of a husband. Despite the stress and fear, this experience was enlightening, motivating me to take action when confronted with injustice.

You can find more about Feminita

on Twitter: @moorlandiya and their website: https://feminita.kz/

Hazel Mead, a 23-year-old activist and illustrator hailing from the UK, has been a pivotal voice in challenging menstrual taboos and promoting period positivity. Hazel was raised with a feeling of shame about her period, even in spite of the UK's generally progressive attitude. This uneasiness resulted from euphemistic language that concealed menstruation's natural occurrence and a lack of candid conversations about it in schools.

Reflecting on her journey, Hazel noted how she discreetly handled period days, concealing pads up her sleeve or ensuring she had pockets available. Determined to spark conversations and normalise discussions about periods, Hazel turned to illustration. Early in her career, she created satirical pieces addressing the tampon tax issue after participating in the #FreePeriods protest.

Hazel actively contributes her drawing abilities to organisations such as Bloody Good Period, which is in line with their objective of offering period products to homeless and asylum seekers. She also participated in Freda's campaign, advocating for the provision of free period products in hotels, schools, airlines, and offices.

Hazel has embraced a more open approach to discussing periods in her personal life. She no longer uses euphemisms and opts for the term 'period products' instead of 'sanitary products,' challenging the implication of uncleanness associated with menstruation.

Although Hazel notes that the UK government's recent announcement to offer free period products in secondary schools and colleges is a positive step, she also stresses the continued need to combat injustices and break menstrual taboos. Although she recognises that much work is ahead, Hazel remains optimistic, believing that sustained efforts and advocacy will continue to bring about positive change.

For those interested in Hazel Mead's work and activism, her presence can be found

on Instagram (@hazel.mead), Twitter (@hazelmeadart), and her website (hazelmead.com).

Samikshya Koirala, a 21-year-old youth executive affiliated with Amnesty International Nepal, is actively challenging the cultural norms surrounding menstruation in Nepal. In the country, menstruating girls are often secluded from the sun and men for up to 15 days, with some even being exiled to cattle sheds in practice known as **chhaupadi**.

Reflecting on her own experience, Samikshya recalls being 11 years old when she had her first period. Despite a grand event taking place at home, she was not allowed to participate and was hidden in a dark room at a relative's house. This tradition deeply affected her, leading to tears and a feeling of exclusion.

After being isolated for five days, Samikshya was subject to additional rules when she got back to her family. These included a 19-day kitchen ban and an 11-day ban from touching male family members. She was too shy after the incident to tell her friends why she hadn't been around.

However, a turning point occurred when a group of young women visited her school to educate students about menstruation. This encounter empowered Samikshya and her peers with the knowledge to challenge existing traditions. Though her family initially resisted, she successfully conveyed the importance of adapting to modern menstrual hygiene practices, eliminating restrictions within her family.

As a member of Amnesty International's Student Group at Kathmandu University, Samikshya is actively involved in reshaping perceptions of menstruation on a broader scale. The group utilises various means, such as creating videos, organising rallies, and implementing community programs for both boys and girls in rural areas. Witnessing open discussions about menstrual issues among children brings pride to Samikshya and her colleagues.

Samickshya is dedicated to eradicating superstitions and

altering people's perceptions of menstruation in Nepal. She thinks they are making great strides towards questioning and changing prevailing cultural norms through their efforts. She discusses her experiences and advocacy efforts on

Instagram at @koiralasamikshya2016.

Poulomi Basu, a 36-year-old transmedia artist and activist hailing from India, has a profound personal understanding of the impact of patriarchal norms on women's lives. She was raised in a patriarchal Hindu home where she witnessed firsthand the constrictive use of customs and rituals to subjugate women. When she left home, she realised that many women in similar circumstances do not have this option, and that was the beginning of her journey towards freedom from such control.

During her exploration, Poulomi encountered stories like that of Tula, a 16-year-old from Nepal. Tula, prohibited from household chores during her period, dedicates this time to working as a porter to support her family. Enduring long journeys with heavy loads, she balances her labour with school exams, earning a meager 20 US cents for her efforts. Another narrative unfolded with Lakshmi, a single mother of three in Nepal, who faces exile imposed by her mother-in-law during menstruation. Despite adversity, Lakshmi's determination to protect and provide for her children remains unbroken.

Witnessing the perilous situations women face during childbirth-related exiles, Poulomi took action. She collaborated with Water Aid and initiated the 'To be a Girl' campaign, providing reusable sanitary pads to 130,000 girls across Nepal, India, and parts of Africa. Additionally, through the 'My Body Is Mine' campaign in partnership with Action Aid, Poulomi encourages women to reclaim control over their narratives. She uses powerful art, storytelling, virtual reality films, and community workshops to empower women to speak out against violence, believing in art's transformative ability.

The impact of Poulomi's efforts reached beyond individual stories. By collaborating with Water Aid, she contributed to pressuring the Nepalese government to criminalise chhaupadi in 2018. Notwithstanding this encouraging development, difficulties still exist because the practice is illegal in some areas. Poulomi, who is aware of the significance of her work, keeps up her campaigns to support women's agency and combat violence.

You can follow Poulomi Basu on

Instagram (@poulomi07), Twitter (@poulomibasu), and explore her work on her website: https://www.poulomibasu.com/

Haafizah Bhamjee is a 22-year-old student and youth activist hailing from South Africa. The issue of period poverty is particularly prevalent within university settings, where discussing menstruation and the affordability of sanitary products remains a taboo. As a result, many girls silently endure the dehumanising effects of this situation.

My friends and I started the #WorthBleedingFor campaign in response to this challenge. We want to dispel the myth that attending college is only a luxury available to the wealthy. People from all economic backgrounds are interested in pursuing higher education. Some students face dire circumstances, resorting to sleeping in libraries or relying on donated grocery packs. The lack of access to sanitary pads compounds their challenges.

To address this issue, we advocate for installing sanitary pad dispensers in university bathrooms. Additionally, we have reached out to local government authorities, urging them to provide free pads for girls in schools. Our campaign also focuses on empowering girls to share their experiences openly.

Witnessing the tangible impact of our efforts is incredibly gratifying. While change may be gradual, the momentum is exhilarating. A group of girls has even produced a video highlighting our #WorthBleedingFor campaign and our advocacy work. Knowing that we are making a difference is truly remarkable. (This story was initially featured on The Lily.)

CHHAUPADI

Let's delve into the distressing ritual of Chhaupadi. In some areas of Western Nepal, women and girls experience exile from their homes during menstruation, as a superstition holds that their presence brings misfortune. This archaic practice, known as "chhaupadi," involves coercing them to reside in isolated huts, distant from family and friends. Despite being prohibited in Nepal since 2005, many communities persist in its observance.

ActionAid actively collaborates with local women's groups in Western Nepal to heighten awareness about the detrimental impacts of chhaupadi and its unlawful status. Through engagement with community leaders, religious figures, and local law enforcement, we strive to eradicate this practice. Additionally, our efforts extend to educating young girls on menstrual hygiene and conducting training sessions for women and girls to produce secure, reusable sanitary pads.

So, what precisely is Chhaupadi? In the secluded regions

of remote and mid-western Nepal, adhering to age-old customs, menstruating females face ostracism. They must dwell outside settlements in cowsheds or small huts to avoid supposedly contaminating their family members. **Razen Manandhar**, a former journalist at The Himalayan Times, sheds light on this practice in his blog:

"They firmly believe that women are impure during these 4-5 days each month, and their gods disapprove of women approaching them during this period. Consequently, men enforce the isolation of menstruating women in cramped huts devoid of windows or doors. Men hold the conviction that if menstruating women remain in their homes, tigers may attack them and their herds, or their gods will be displeased, resulting in illness. Astonishingly, they prioritise an unseen deity over their own family members."

In Kailali, Nepal, there stands a modest shed measuring four feet high and four feet wide, known as a "goth," where Durga Buda, aged 31, spends four nights every month. Constructed from bamboo, straw, and wood, its walls are coated with a mixture of mud and cow dung.

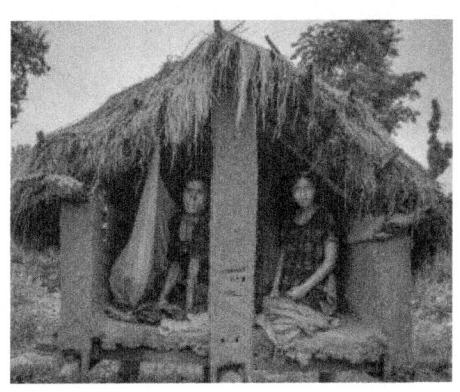

Two girls in a Chhaupadi hut (CrackitTodayAffairs, 2023)

Though accustomed to her routine, Buda admits that the constant fear of encountering wild animals, snakes, and inebriated individuals persists. She relies on a thin, worn wool blanket, bearing frayed edges each night. The mosquito net she sleeps under reveals signs of repair, with some holes carefully stitched and others secured with safety pins.

While her family of eight, including in-laws, sleeps comfortably in a mud-brick house, Buda finds herself relegated to the backyard, situated alongside two cows and six goats. Her seclusion results from adhering to the age-old chaupadi ritual, a prevalent practice in the far and mid-western regions of Nepal. This tradition dictates that women must be isolated to a cowshed, hut, barn, or cave during menstruation and childbirth, as they are believed to carry impurity that can bring misfortune to the family, neighbours, and domestic animals.

Reflecting on her initial experience during her first period, Buda recalls being segregated for a daunting 11 days. "I was scared, cold, and confused, but the fear of sin prevailed," she states. This Hindu tradition transcends caste boundaries in the region and is deeply rooted in Hinduism. Women who defy this practice are held responsible for crop failures, illnesses, and sudden deaths among animals. Buda, echoing the sentiment of many, questions, "Who wants to be ostracized?" (Das, 2014).

A Nepali teenager, aged 16, has lost her life due to the illegal tradition of Chhaupadi, where menstruating women are compelled to reside in makeshift huts outside their homes. Anita Chand, hailing from the Baitadi district in the western part of the country near the Indian border, reportedly succumbed to a snake bite while sleeping. This marks the first reported fatality linked to Chhaupadi since 2019, raising concerns among advocates who fear setbacks in efforts to eradicate this practice.

Chhaupadi, prohibited since 2005, carries penalties of up to three months imprisonment and a fine of 3,000 Nepalese rupees (approximately 20 euros). Authorities in the Baitadi district are currently investigating Anita's demise, with her family refuting claims that she was menstruating at the time of her death.

Bina Bhatta, the vice president of Baitadi's Pancheshwar Rural Municipality, underlined the continuous efforts to put an end to Chhaupadi but also acknowledged the significant amount of work that remains. The most recent known death connected to Chhaupadi happened in 2019, when 21-year-old Parwati Budha Rawat passed away after staying three nights in an outdoor hut. This incident prompted nationwide programs and campaigns to eliminate the practice, destroying thousands of period huts. However, recent reports suggest a resurgence in the construction of these huts.

Pashupati Kunwar, a campaigner against Chhaupadi for 25 years, highlighted the destruction of over 7,000 period huts in the district following Parwati's death. However, the focus shifted during the COVID-19 pandemic, leading to decreased efforts to combat Chhaupadi. Radha Paudel, founder of the Global South Coalition for Dignified Menstruation, criticised the Nepalese government for insufficient implementation of laws and policies aimed at preventing the expulsion of women during their periods.

While ActionAid successfully eliminated Chhaupadi from 11 communities in Western Nepal, further concerted efforts are required for women to assert their rights and openly oppose such harmful practices.

EPILOGUE

"In the grand tapestry of existence, diversity is the vibrant thread that weaves the narrative of strength. Embrace the multitude of perspectives, for in the mosaic of differences, we find the resilience of a civilization's soul." -
Friedrich Nietzsche.

Coming to the end of this exploration into the complex world of the vagina, and having travelled through the myths, prejudices and misconceptions; the harsh realities surrounding menstruation; and the worrisome practice of female genital mutilation (FGM), one thing becomes apparent. This journey was not simply meant to uncover the mysteries behind social taboos, but more importantly to foster a deeper understanding, appreciation and empathy.

As I reflect on the knowledge that came to light, through the research, stories and anecdotes I shared with you, it is clear to me that my mission which initially aimed at unravelling unsettling truths, gradually transformed into a manifesto, cultivating an optimistic outlook.

The exlopration began with the recognition that the vagina, more so than any other part of the female body, has been surrounded in myth, superstition and fear throughout history. From ancient beliefs to modern urban legends, the narrative is often secluded in a haze of mystery, often fueled by societal dysphoria. Nevertheless, by fostering education, encouraging open dialogue and dismantling misconceptions, both women and men can become empowered to adopt a more enlightened perspective.

On this journey I continued to travel through the vast landscape of prejudices on questioning social norms that have burdened people's consciousness globally. Though I soon realised that questioning can only be fruitful when accompanied by uncensored communication and informed debate, challenging and dismantling stigmas. Only then can people trully celebrate the diversity of their experiences and the uniqueness of their bodies, free from the constraints of societal judgment.

It is evident that social expectations, cultural norms and gender biases have contributed immensely to the perpetuation of such harmful stereotypes. Thus, navigating this complex terrain helped set a new goal, beyond the disassembling of all kinds of barriers; to promote a more comprehensive and informed understanding of the diversity and complexity inherent in women's experiences.

Examining menstruation, a natural and integral part of billions of women's lives, revealed the stigmas and challenges faced by those who menstruate. From period poverty to the normalisation of menstruation as a natural bodily function, it is our collective responsibility to cast aside the anchors that prevent open conversations and access to necessary resources.

The darkest corner of the exploration brought me face to face with the abhorrent practice of female genital mutilation. This tradition, deeply rooted into culture has left its mark on countless women, both physically and emotionally. By shedding light on the reality of FGM, I hope to have contributed to the ongoing global efforts to eradicate this violation of human rights, to protect vulnerable individuals, and to promote true gender equality.

As I close the pages of this book, let the thought be impressed upon us that knowledge is a powerful force for change. By dispelling toxic myths, challenging prejudices and encouraging understanding, we can pave the way for a future where narratives around the vagina are free of ignorance, discrimination, and pain, physical and mental.

In this collective journey toward enlightenment, I would like to invite you to let empathy be your guide and may the voices of those whose stories have been shared in these pages resonate, encouraging us all to create a world that celebrates strength, resilience and the beuty inherent in every individual.

REFERENCE LIST

Abathun, A.D., Sundby, J. and Gele, A.A. (2016) "Attitude toward female genital mutilation among Somali and Harari people, Eastern Ethiopia", *International journal of women's health*, pp.557-569. doi: 10.2147%2FIJWH.S112226.

Abdulcadir J, Guedj NS, Yaron M, et al. (2022) *Female Genital Mutilation/Cutting in Children and Adolescents: Illustrated Guide to Diagnose, Assess, Inform and Report* [Internet]. Cham (CH): Springer, Chapter 5. Available from: https://www.ncbi.nlm.nih.gov/books/NBK592359/ doi: 10.1007/978-3-030-81736-7_5

(Accessed: January 15, 2024).

Abebe, S., Dessalegn, M., Hailu, Y. and Makonnen, M. (2020) "Prevalence and barriers to ending female genital cutting: The case of Afar and Amhara regions of Ethiopia", *International Journal of Environmental Research and Public Health*, 17(21), p. 7960. doi:10.3390/ijerph17217960.

Action Aid. (2016) *Female genital mutilation (FGM), ActionAid*

UK. Available at: https://www.actionaid.org.uk/our-work/vawg/female-genital-mutilation (Accessed: January 19, 2024).

Baral, M. (2018) *Success Story Of The Real 'Padman'; From A School Dropout To A Social Entrepreneur*. Available at: https://www.ndtv.com/education/success-story-of-the-real-padman-from-a-school-dropout-to-a-social-entrepreneur-1791399 (Accessed: January 15, 2024).

Boyden, J. (2013) *Harmful traditional practices and child protection: Contested understandings and practices of female child marriage and circumcision in Ethiopia*. Oxford, UK: Young Lives.

Brooklyn Museum, B.M. (no date) *The Dinner Party by Judy Chicago, Brooklyn Museum*. Available at: https://www.brooklynmuseum.org/exhibitions/dinner_party/ (Accessed: 09 December 2023).

Center for Urologic Care of Berks County. (year unknown) *Kegel exercises*. Available at: https://www.centerforurologiccare.com/patient-education/kegel-exercises/ (Accessed: January 18, 2024).

Cokal, S. (2018) *Clean porn: Hot sex and hair removal*, *Medium*.

Available at: https://cokal.medium.com/clean-porn-the-visual-aesthetics-of-hygiene-hot-sex-and-hair-removal-ac188fc9161d (Accessed: January 11, 2024).

Connor, L. (2022) *Most voters back our campaign to end period poverty in UK - here are our demands, The Mirror*. Available at: https://www.mirror.co.uk/news/uk-news/most-voters-back-campaign-end-28417685 (Accessed: January 15, 2024).

Das, B. (2014) *Nepal's menstrual exiles, Al Jazeera*. Available at: https://www.aljazeera.com/features/2014/2/10/nepals-menstrual-exiles (Accessed: January 17, 2024).

Elamin, W., and A.J. Mason-Jones. (2020) "Female Genital Mutilation/Cutting: A Systematic Review and Meta-Ethnography Exploring Women's Views of Why It Exists and Persists." *International Journal of Sexual Health*, 32(1), pp.1–21.

Equality Now. (2020) Aisha – Singapore. Available at: https://equalitynow.org/stories/aisha-singapore/ (Accessed: January 18, 2024).

Gipson, F. (2020) *Art Matters podcast: the Vagina Museum and vulvas in art* (no date) *Artuk.org*. Available at: https://artuk.org/discover/stories/art-matters-podcast-the-vagina-museum-and-vulvas-in-art (Accessed: January 19, 2024).

Gunter, J. (2019) *The vagina bible: The Vulva and the vagina - separating the myth from the medicine.* London: Piatkus.

Johnston, A. (2019) "I visited the world's first Vagina Museum, and the gift shop was the highlight," *Business Insider*, 25 November. Available at: https://www.businessinsider.com/photos-inside-worlds-first-vagina-museum-london-england-2019-11 (Accessed: January 19, 2024).

Kearl, J. (2021) *Maryum saifee: Foreign service officer, women's rights activist, & FGM survivor, Utahglobaldiplomacy.org*. Utah Global Diplomacy. Available at: https://utahglobaldiplomacy.org/friends-of-utah-avena-prince/item/399-maryum-saifee-foreign-service-officer-women-s-rights-activist-fgm-survivor (Accessed: January 15, 2024).

Kendall, P. (2014) *Here's that 'Vagina kayak' Japanese artist Megumi Igarashi made with the help of crowdfunding*, RocketNews24. Available at: https://web.archive.org/web/20161104044743/http://en.rocketnews24.com/2014/07/18/heres-that-vagina-kayak-japanese-artist-megumi-igarashi-made-with-the-help-of-crowdfunding/ (Accessed: 09 December 2023).

Lawford, E. (2023) *The biologist behind the vagina museum, Prospect Magazine - Britain's leading monthly current affairs magazine.* Available at: https://www.prospectmagazine.co.uk/views/people/63741/the-biologist-behind-the-vagina-museum (Accessed: 09 December 2023).

Lidell, H., Scott, R. and Konstantinidou, A. (no date) *Mega Lexicon of the Greek language.*

Mehari, G., Molla, A., Mamo, A., & Matanda, D. (2020) Exploring changes in female genital mutilation/cutting: shifting norms and practices among communities in Fafan and West Arsi zones, Ethiopia. Evidence to End FGM/C: Research to Help Girls and Women Thrive. New York: Population Council.

Menstrupedia. (2024) Menstrupedia. Available at: https://www.menstrupedia.com/ (Accessed: January 15, 2024).

NHS. (2022) National Health Service: Overview -Female genital mutilation (FGM). Available at: https://www.nhs.uk/conditions/female-genital-mutilation-fgm/ (Accessed: January 15, 2024).

Prof Wilson. (2021) Vaginoplasty/ Vulvoplasty/ Labiaplasty/

vaginal tightening. Available at: https://prof-wilson.com/vaginoplasty-vulvoplasty-labiaplasty-vaginal-tightening/ (Accessed: January 18, 2024).

QR Code Generator pro. (No date) Available at: https://app.qr-code-generator.com (Accessed: January 25, 2024).

Quartz Clinique. (2023) *Vulvoplasty*. Available at: https://www.quartzclinique.com/en/vulvoplasty (Accessed: January 18, 2024).

Real Styling Solutions. (2022) *What is Vaginal Bleaching and Anal Bleaching*. Available at: https://www.realstylingsolutions.com/what-is-vaginal-bleaching-and-anal-bleaching/ (Accessed: January 18, 2024).

Ruitenbeek, H. M. (1966) *Psychoanalysis and male sexuality*. Lanham, MD: Rowman & Littlefield.

Saatchi Art. (2022) *Vulva 240 sculpture*. Available at: https://www.saatchiart.com/art/Sculpture-Vulva-240/1824604/10837299/view (Accessed: January 12, 2024).

The great wall of vulva. (2024) *Plaster casts of 400 people's genitals*. Available at: https://www.thegreatwallofvulva.com/ (Accessed: January 15, 2024).

The Live Life. (2021) *FGM and

female cutting: The facts. Available at: https://thelivelifecouk.wordpress.com/2021/06/02/fgm-and-female-cutting-the-facts/ (Accessed: January 15, 2024).

The London Free Press. (2014) *Vagina kayak artist arrested again in Japan.* Available at: https://lfpress.com/2014/12/03/japanese-woman-arrested-again-over-genitals-art-work (Accessed: January 15, 2024)

The Mysterious Venus of Willendorf. (2022) *The Collector.* Available at: https://www.thecollector.com/venus-of-willendorf/ (Accessed: January 16, 2024).

The Stone Yoni. (year unknown) *By Binh Giang - self-taken at the National Museum of Vietnam History.* Available at: https://commons.wikimedia.org/w/index.php?curid=2889577 (Acceced: January 15, 2024).

UNICEF. (2019) *Female genital mutilation (FGM) statistics.* Available at: https://data.unicef.org/topic/child-protection/female-genital-mutilation/ (Accessed: January 10, 2024).

Unknown. (2023) *Chhaupadi : Period Hut Ritual Of Nepal, Crackit Today Affairs.* Available at: https://crackittoday.com/current-affairs/chhaupadi-period-hut-ritual-of-nepal/ (Accessed: January 14, 2024).

USAID. (2021) *Purity's story, U.S. Agency for International Development*. Available at: https://medium.com/usaid-2030/puritys-story-855e6f83234c (Accessed: January 17, 2024).

Varma, A. (2023) *Abiding or autonomous? The dangers of female genital mutilation, Leveled Legislation*. Available at: https://medium.com/leveled-legislation/abiding-or-autonomous-the-dangers-of-female-genital-mutilation-9432ca65359d (Accessed: January 17, 2024).

Wamsley, L. (2020) "Scotland poised to become 1st country to make period products free," *NPR*, 27 February. Available at: https://www.npr.org/sections/goatsandsoda/2020/02/27/809990550/scotland-poised-to-become-1st-country-to-make-period-products-free (Accessed: January 19, 2024).

Wateraid. (2021) *Why celebrities and activists are wearing period bracelets this Menstrual Hygiene Day*. Available at: https://www.wateraid.org/uk/blog/period-bracelets (Accessed: January 10, 2024).

Waterlow, L. (2015) *Kenyan teen reveals how she was forced to undergo female genital mutilation*. Available at: https://www.dailymail.co.uk/femail/article-3187784/Teenager-reveals-forced-undergo-female-genital-mutilation-married-man-TWICE-age.html (Accessed: January 15, 2024).

Waxwax. (2023) *What is A Brazilian wax? The ultimate guide.* Available at: https://waxwax.com/brazilian-wax/ (Accessed: January 11, 2024).

Wayne. (2013) Janus, God of the Threshold. Available at:https://ferrebeekeeper.wordpress.com/2013/05/16/janus-god-of-the-threshold/ (Accessed: January 12, 2024).

Weiss-Wolf,J. (2017) *Periods Gone Public: Taking a Stand for Menstrual Equity.* Arcade Publishing, NY.

AFTERWORD

These were The Vagina Chronicles; not just a book, but a movement, a celebration of diversity and a call to embrace the power within. Whether you sought to challenge preconceived notions, to embark on a journey of self-exploration, or to simply expand your understanding of what it means to be a woman, this engaging guide was meant to enlighten, inspire, and empower you.

Let the Chronicles be your companion in your search for the truth, liberation, and celebration of the amazing journey that is womanhood. May this journey spark conversations, challenge preconceptions, and drive the force of change in generations to come.

ABOUT THE AUTHOR

Betty Iliadis

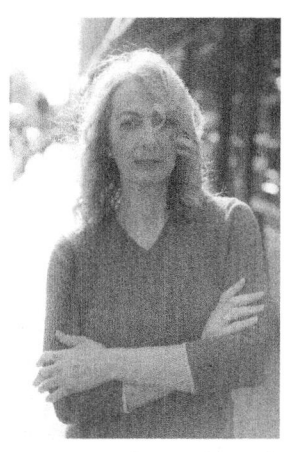

Through her journey in the realms of law, psychology and activism, the author of The Vagina Chronicles has not only mastered the intricacies of the legal system, but has also deved into the complexities of the human mind, understanding the nuanced interplay between law and psychology in the pursuit of justice. Certified by Harvard University in the field of the protection of children's rights, she aspires to create a world where justice in not just a legal concept, but a lived reality for all.

An activist, and member of UN Women UK, she invites for a global dialogue on women's rights and gender equality. In addition, she is a new writer member of the SWWJ, an organisation that promotes women's voices in literature and journalism. Betty Iliadis' journey is not just a personal triumph, it is a testament to the transofrmative power of knowledge and empathy, driven by the unwavering commitment to making the world a better, safer, more inclusive place.

Printed in Great Britain
by Amazon